RECIPES FOR HEALTH

Irritable Bowel Syndrome

RECIPES FOR HEALTH

Irritable Bowel Syndrome

Over 100 recipes for coping with this digestive disorder

ANN PAGE-WOOD AND JILL DAVIES

Thorsons
An Imprint of HarperCollins*Publishers*

Thorsons
An Imprint of HarperCollins*Publishers*
77–85 Fulham Palace Road,
Hammersmith, London W6 8JB
1160 Battery Street,
San Francisco, California 94111–1213

First published by Thorsons as Special Diet Cookbook:
Irritable Bowel Syndrome 1991
This edition 1995
1 3 5 7 9 10 8 6 4 2

A CIP catalogue record for this book
is available from the British Library

ISBN 0 7225 3141-9

Typeset by
Harper Phototypesetters Limited, Northampton
Printed in Great Britain by
The Bath Press, Bath, Avon

Contents

Foreword

THE 'IRRITABLE BOWEL SYNDROME' (IBS) is a troublesome, sometimes distressing condition which is often painful and affects more women than men. The cause of the condition is at present obscure. In different individuals and even in the same individual, cramping pain is often accompanied by altered bowel habit which may vary with diarrhoea fluctuating with constipation and flatulence. It is a feature of this disorder that careful investigation shows no evidence of a physical cause. Changes in diet, particularly an increase in 'fibre' intake, may decrease the severity of symptoms and enable sufferers to pursue reasonably normal lives.

For all those who suffer from IBS, the second edition of this book, like the first, is a truly practical guide. It starts with a useful outline of facts about the disease, proceeding to a discussion of its holistic management. The entire book has been updated to include new advances in our understanding of the condition. The main bulk of the book provides dietary guidelines with a selection of tried and tested recipes to suit a variety of tastes and clinical problems. Following the advice provided in the book will enable IBS sufferers to have a varied diet and at the same time meet the principal dietary requirement of increasing the intake of what is commonly called 'dietary fibre' or simply 'roughage'.

The value of this book is greatly increased by the experience and interest of the authors in the disease.

J.W.T. Dickerson
Emeritus Professor of
Human Nutrition

Facts about irritable bowel syndrome

WHO SUFFERS FROM IRRITABLE BOWEL SYNDROME?

Irritable bowel syndrome (IBS) is believed to affect about one third of the population in the United Kingdom. It is the most common condition seen in gastroenterology outpatient clinics with over 50 per cent of the patients there suffering from its effects. It is difficult to determine at what age the condition develops because people have often had symptoms for many years before seeking help, but patients most frequently seek medical advice between the ages of 20 and 40.

The disorder is more common in women than in men and has been well recognized for more than 150 years. In 1849 one medical practitioner noted that it was '. . . so common that it can scarcely have failed to obtrude itself on the notice of every practitioner'.

WHAT IS IRRITABLE BOWEL SYNDROME?

Over 50 terms have been used in English literature to describe the condition that we now refer to as Irritable Bowel Syndrome. Some of the different names used include: spastic colon, mucous colitis, mucomembranous colitis, non-inflammatory colitis, stress colitis, irritable gut syndrome, irritable colon, irritated bowel syndrome. We may well ask 'What's in a name?', but it is important because some of the terms used are misleading. The classic example of this is the term 'mucous colitis'. This is rather unfortunate because excess mucus production is not reported by all IBS patients. Moreover the word 'colitis' implies inflammation and there is no evidence of inflammation in IBS.

WHAT ARE THE SYMPTOMS OF IRRITABLE BOWEL SYNDROME?

Patients with IBS often complain of a variety of symptoms (in medical terms, a 'symptom complex' rather than a 'single homogeneous syndrome').

As one frustrated sufferer is reported to have said, 'If you have to live with gut ache like this, you can't be doing with a doctor who thinks you're imagining it'.

The major symptoms associated with IBS are:

- abdominal pain
- variable bowel habit (constipation/diarrhoea)
- abdominal distension (bloating)

- pain relief with defecation
- frequent and loose stools with pain
- excess mucus in stools
- sensation of incomplete evacuation.

Abdominal pain

This is one of the major features of IBS and is usually the reason patients initially consult a doctor. The pain may occur anywhere in the abdomen, either at a single or multiple sites (see Figure 1).

It is rare for the pain to occur outside the abdomen although it is sometimes felt in the back. The pain is described as aching, colicky or cramp-like; it may be mild or severe and is typically intermittent and relapsing in nature. It may last for a few minutes or many hours but it rarely lasts for more than 24 hours and does not wake the patient from sleep. The pain is often brought on by a meal, particularly breakfast, and is frequently relieved by defecation or the passing of wind.

Altered Bowel Habit

This is found in the majority of patients. The alterations may be intermittent or continuous and may be either constipation or diarrhoea or, characteristically, alternating constipation and diarrhoea.

Abdominal Distension (bloating)

This is common in IBS. The distension is usually at its worst in the evening.

Flatulence, which tends to result in unpleasant

rumblings in the bowel or the passing of wind, is also a frequent symptom.

Mucus in Stools

This is frequently reported by IBS patients. Mucus is the natural lubricant of the digestive tract. Many IBS patients are certainly conscious of passing more mucus than usual.

Other Symptoms

IBS patients have more than their fair share of nausea, vomiting, dyspepsia, migraine and other forms of headache, fatigue, frequency and urgency of passing urine and, in females, painful menstruation.

WHAT CAN TRIGGER THE SYMPTOMS OF IBS?

So much for the symptoms of IBS, but what precisely is irritable bowel syndrome and what causes it? These may sound surprising questions, but the answers are uncertain. In the words of a highly respected gastroenterologist, 'the underlying disorder remains unknown so . . . hypotheses abound and opinions vary, depending on current medical fashion and the personal preference of the clinical investigator'. A look at research into the subject, however, helps to give a general insight into the nature of IBS and factors that are associated with the onset of symptoms. This is very important with regard to managing the condition. A 'good' manager has to know what he or she is dealing with.

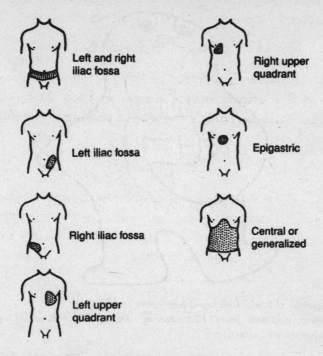

Figure 1 Sites of pain in irritable bowel syndrome.
Source: 'Prognosis in the irritable bowel syndrome: a 5-year prospective study' by R.F. Harvey, E.C. Maud and A.M. Brown in *The Lancet*, page 963, 25 April, 1987.

IBS is universally accepted as a disorder of 'gastro-intestinal motor activity'. In simple terms IBS patients have a more sensitive gut and this makes the colon contract too strongly.

Factors that may trigger IBS symptoms are outlined below:

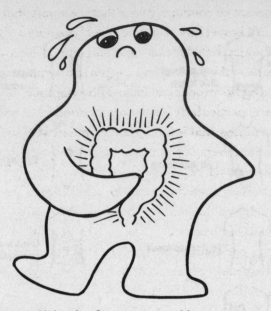

Figure 2   Irritable bowel syndrome – more sensitive gut
Source: Adapted from *Understanding your Irritable Bowel* (Duphar Laboratories Limited).

- **meal patterns** are probably an important consideration. Missing meals and snacking as a substitute will have implications for gut function
- **specific foods** might exacerbate symptoms
- **dietary fibre deficiency** could be a contributory factor in some cases, as lack of fibre may predispose towards constipation
- **fat** may be a trigger in some IBS patients as the fatty acids in fat stimulate the release of a hormone called cholecystokinin – a potent stimulant of colonic motor activity

- **drugs** are so commonly used that their potential to disturb bowel function should not be ignored. Antacids, antibiotics, beta blockers and narcotics all have adverse effects on the gut that can trigger IBS symptoms
- **ovarian hormones** can make IBS symptoms more severe, particularly just before a period
- **gastrointestinal infections** may initiate IBS symptoms. Some sufferers can pinpoint that their symptoms began with an attack of gastroenteritis
- **abdominal operations** may be significant as studies have shown that many IBS patients have had appendicectomies
- **stress, personality and psyche** Psychological factors probably accentuate an underlying predisposition to the condition.

HOW DO YOU KNOW IF YOU HAVE IBS?

The non-specific nature of irritable bowel syndrome makes clinical diagnosis very important. No matter how tempting it is to self-diagnose, it is essential that the diagnosis is left to the experts. However, patients can help in this process simply by making some notes about their symptoms and taking them along to their doctor. Just as we like to have a 'good' doctor, equally, doctors appreciate 'good' patients. If you can give your doctor an accurate medical history, one that is clear with the onset of the various symptoms in the correct time sequence, this will greatly help the doctor as these details play an important part in the diagnosis.

Facts about irritable bowel syndrome

If you suspect that you suffer from IBS, you should first consult your doctor. Diagnosis can be made from a medical history, physical examination and some diagnostic tests.

A high percentage of IBS patients fear that they may have cancer before they are diagnosed as having IBS. This is understandable, because two of the symptoms of IBS, namely diarrhoea and/or constipation, are, indeed, also associated with carcinoma and polyps. Some of the symptoms also overlap with other disorders. For example, diarrhoea and/or constipation are also associated with inflammatory bowel disease, chronic intestinal infection and coeliac disease. Similarly, upper abdominal pain is also an indication of peptic ulceration, gallstones and chronic pancreatitis. So, you can see, it is important not to speculate. The need for a confident diagnosis by the experts cannot be too strongly emphasized.

2

Management of
irritable bowel syndrome

ONCE IBS HAS been diagnosed, your doctor should reassure you about the nature of the disorder and give you specific management strategies. Probably the most important thing your doctor can do for you is reassure you as just knowing that there is no serious disease of the colon helps a lot. IBS may well cause discomfort, but it will not shorten your life, nor does it lead to any other disease. Treatment is directed towards relieving the symptoms and identifying factors that possibly exacerbate the condition.

Treatment of IBS will of course be tailored to your own particular circumstances with the aim to relieve symptoms. *Diet* is a key issue, as indicated by the title of this book, but pharmacological preparations and a range of alternative therapies may also be prescribed.

MEDICALLY PRESCRIBED TREATMENTS

Before discussing various preparations that might be prescribed, it is interesting to note medical opinion on the use of drugs for the treatment of IBS. It is accepted that:

- drugs can't cure the condition, but they can ease the symptoms
- drugs should be used sparingly to avoid the possibility of becoming dependent on them
- any drug therapy should not be harmful or associated with serious side effects.

Bulking agents speed the passage of contents through the colon, resulting in softer, bulkier stools. Because of this action, they are sometimes prescribed for those IBS sufferers who experience pain from either constipation or the frequent passage of pellety stools.

Until recently, most gastroenterologists considered bran worth a try. However, attitudes on the use of bran are changing as a result of scentific studies on IBS patients. Other bulking agents to choose from are shown.

Figure 3   Bulking agents

Substance	Brand name
Ispaghula	Fybogel Regulan Isogel Metamucil Vi-siblin
Sterculia	Normacol Inolaxine
Methylcellulose	Celevac Cellucon Cologel

The use of laxatives is a controversial issue and medical opinion varies on their use for IBS. Some medical practitioners never prescribe laxatives for the condition while others give their patients small, regular doses of either senna or lactulose that stimulate the bowel, keeping its contents moving and therefore soft.

Drugs that stop diarrhoea may be of benefit to some patients whose main symptom is persistent diarrhoea. Examples of these drugs include codeine phosphate, diphenoxylate and loperamide. Codeine phosphate is perhaps the least desirable choice as it can be addictive if used over a long period of time in high doses. Diphenoxylate and loperamide are effective, with fewer side-effects being found with loperamide.

Antispasmodics are sometimes prescribed for the treatment of IBS and work, as their name suggests, to reduce the spasm in the colon. Examples of the drugs most commonly used include propantheline (Pro-Banthine), hyoscine (Buscopan), dicyclomine (Merbentyl), mebeverine (Colofac) and peppermint oil (Colpermin).

Some specialists prescribe mild tranquillizers intermittently, for example, valium and ativan. It is generally believed that these are best avoided due to the risk of dependency. They would normally be prescribed for short-term use if there was an acutely stressful situation.

Some doctors feel strongly that antidepressants or mood elevating drugs help their patients, but care needs to be taken in the selection as they can cause an increase in constipation.

Interestingly, drug combinations have proved successful

in the treatment of IBS. Due to the complexity of the disorder, no one drug can be expected to have a lasting broad-spectrum effect. One recent study found that a combination of mebeverine, Fybogel and Motival relieved the symptoms in most of the patients.

ALTERNATIVE THERAPIES

Before discussing various alternative therapies and certainly before you go to receive alternative treatment, think carefully about the following:

- anxiety and depression are to be expected if you have suffered for long periods with little in the way of successful treatment and, as is sometimes the case, little sympathy from your doctor
- some anxieties will be allayed by the investigation itself
- emotional pressures can sometimes be relieved by discussion
- changes to lifestyle and behaviour may make all the difference – is breakfast a hasty scramble? is lunch a sandwich gulped down while the telephone is ringing?

Psychotherapy

This can be useful in the management of IBS. It has been shown that patients who had attended ten one hour individual psychotherapy sessions over three months, combined with drug therapy, showed greater improvement than patients receiving only drugs.

Psychiatric therapy

This is rarely necessary as psychiatrists can only be expected to help those with IBS if they have psychiatric problems.

Hypnotherapy

IBS patients may have this prescribed for them. This form of treatment is increasing in popularity but it is very time-consuming and expensive.

Meditation, relaxation and biofeedback techniques

Not enough research has been carried out into these methods to give a confident appraisal of their benefits. If you do choose one of these therapies, however, it is important that you see a suitably qualified person. You are most likely to find these types of treatment attractive if you prefer it to focus on your symptoms rather than on any emotional dimension of your condition.

DIET

Diet is, without doubt, a key factor in the management of IBS. Recently it was found that when patients were asked what advice they would pass on to others with the disorder, many clearly regarded diet as the most important aspect of their long-term treatment. Here are some general guidelines about diet and how it can affect the symptoms of IBS.

- **Size and timing of meals** Snacking in place of meals should be avoided. Meals should be eaten regularly, to include breakfast, midday and evening meals.
- **Foods** Certain foods may trigger the symptoms of IBS. Make a note of those which seem to make the condition worse, but consult your doctor before eliminating these foods altogether. Many sufferers of IBS eliminate so many foods that they end up eating 'unbalanced' meals. The fear of eating specific foods can be carried too far and may lead to a deficient diet.
- **Excessive coffee and tea** intake is not advisable if you are suffering from diarrhoea, as the caffeine stimulates bowel action. Some patients, particularly those with diarrhoea, also find that their symptoms are brought on by milk and its products. These patients probably also have alactasia, a condition that impairs the absorption of lactose (the kind of sugar found in milk) and when lactose reaches the colon it has a laxative effect. It is important that these patients avoid milk and any of its products, but check this with your doctor first.
- **Dietary fibre** Throughout the book, the term fibre has been used to refer to dietary fibre. Dietary fibre is of vegetable origin and differs from the fibres found in animal foods such as meat or fish. IBS sufferers who are constipated (e.g. less than three bowel actions a week, the need to strain at defecation, production of compact/pellety stools) may benefit from an increase in the fibre content of their diet.
- **Fat** A reduction in fat intake may be of benefit if you

suffer pain after meals. Avoiding rich dishes and excess fat should minimize the release of cholecystokinin that, as we noted before, stimulates the colon.

3

Dietary guidelines for irritable bowel syndrome

WHAT DO THE dietary recommendations mean? How can they be implemented? Here are some straightforward principles to make the recommendations part of your everyday life.

- Eat regularly and avoid snacking and binges – include breakfast, midday and evening meals.
- To ensure that you eat a healthy diet, choose foods at each meal following the meal-planning scheme below.
- Avoid 'offending' foods in consultation with your doctor.
- If you suffer from constipation choose food that will increase the amount of fibre in your diet (see pages 18–21).
- Cut down the amount of fat in your diet (see pages 21–23).
- Cut down on your intake of caffeinated drinks such as tea and coffee.

HOW DO I MAKE SURE I EAT
A HEALTHY DIET?

To ensure that the balance is right, select foods at each meal from each of the following groups: *rich sources of protein, cereals*, preferably unrefined, and *fruit* or *vegetables* (see Fig. 4).

Figure 4 Meal-planning scheme

Protein-rich	Meat, poultry, offal, fish, eggs, milk, cheese, yogurt, pulses, nuts.
Cereals	Wholemeal bread, crispbread, wholemeal pasta, brown rice, breakfast cereals.
Fruit and vegetables	Apples, oranges, bananas, tomatoes, avocado pears, carrots, potatoes, cauliflower.

The recipe section has been divided into three main parts along these lines to show you how the scheme works. The individual recipes have been designed to keep the levels of added fat, sugar and salt to a minimum so that they are in line with healthy eating guidelines.

The advantage of this scheme is that others can enjoy the same food as you, the IBS patient. This puts less of a burden on the cook as preparing different meals for just one individual that are different from the rest of the family is very time-consuming.

HOW DO I INCREASE THE FIBRE IN MY DIET?

Dietary fibre is only found in foods of plant origin – there are lots of things you can do to increase the amount of fibre in your diet. A glance at the recipes will give you a general insight into this.

- Be sure to include a food from the cereal group at every meal (see Figure 4, page 17).
- Eat wholemeal bread in preference to white bread (see Table 1) and use it as an ingredient, for example, toppings, coatings and stuffings.
- Substitute wholemeal pasta for white (see Table 1) or flavoured varieties. Remember to allow for the slightly longer time wholemeal pasta takes to cook.
- Choose brown rice rather than white (see Table 1), simply allow extra cooking time.
- Opt for high-fibre varieties of crispbread rather than crackers and oatcakes.
- Use wholemeal flour in preference to white flour when preparing flour-based dishes. If necessary compromise and use brown flour or half white and half wholemeal flour.
- Select high-fibre breakfast cereals (see Table 2, page 20) rather than fibre-depleted varieties. A hearty bowl of cereal may well fill the 'fibre gap' and breakfast cereals can be used at times other than breakfast, such as toppings, coatings and fillers in burgers and meat loaves.

TABLE 1   UNREFINED CEREALS VERSUS REFINED CEREALS

	Unrefined	Refined	Dietary fibre (g/100g)
Bread	wholemeal,		5.8
	brown		3.5
		white	1.5
Pasta	wholemeal, boiled		3.5
		white, boiled	1.2
Rice	brown, boiled		0.8
		white, boiled	0.2

Source 'Cereals and Cereal Products', the third supplement to McCance Widdowson's *The Composition of Foods* (4th Edition), B. Holland, I.D. Unwin and D.H. Buss, Royal Society of Chemistry, 1988.

- Choose pulse dishes such as baked beans, hummus, lentil soup and tofu burgers as the protein-rich component of meals as a change from meat or fish.
- Include fruit or vegetables or, better still, both, in each meal. Only remove the skins if necessary and leave the vegetables in soups and sauces 'chunky' or liquidize but do not pass the mixtures through a sieve otherwise you will be throwing away valuable fibre.

TABLE 2 BREAKFAST CEREALS PROVIDING A USEFUL SOURCE OF DIETARY FIBRE

Cereal variety	Dietary fibre (g/100g)
All-Bran	24.5
Bran Buds	20.0
Bran Flakes	11.3
Sultana Bran	10.0
Shredded Wheat	9.8
Weetabix	9.7
Shreddies	9.5
Fruit 'n' Fibre	7.0

Source 'Cereals and Cereal Products', the third supplement to McCance Widdowson's *The Composition of Foods* (4th Edition) B. Holland, I.D. Unwin and D.H. Buss, Royal Society of Chemistry, 1988.

- To satisfy a 'sweet tooth', try fresh fruit or dried fruit as an alternative to sweets or chocolate.
- If puddings are on the menu, choose fresh fruit salad, a wholemeal-based bread pudding, fruit with wholemeal toppings or high-fibre cakes rather than mousses, soufflés and milk puddings, which contain little or no fibre.

HOW MUCH FIBRE SHOULD I AIM TO EAT?

Average daily intakes of dietary fibre in the U.K. diet are around 13 grams. Intakes of less than 12 grams are associated with increased risk of bowel disease. The

Department of Health has proposed that adult diets should contain an average for the population of 18 grams per day from a variety of foods whose constituents contain it as a naturally integrated component. If our meal-planning scheme, taking on board the ways of increasing your fibre intake, is followed, this figure is achievable. An alternative approach would be to monitor your fibre intake and note when you can produce soft stools without straining. This will be your optimum intake.

HOW CAN YOU REDUCE THE FAT IN YOUR DIET?

Foods such as butter, margarine, cream and the fat on meat are obviously 'fatty' and so, logically, are called 'visible fat'. Other foods contain fat but this may be less obvious, for example, cakes, biscuits and pastries. These fats are described as 'invisible'. To decrease the amount of fat in your diet there are a lot of things you can do. A quick look at the recipe section should enlighten you on this as reducing fat content was an important consideration in the design of the recipes, but here are a few general pointers.

- **Meat** contributes about 25 per cent of the fat in the diet. Choose lean rather than fatty meat and buy sausages with reduced fat content rather than full-fat varieties. Trim any visible fat from meat and, after cooking stews and casseroles, remove any fat that floats to the surface. Opt for poultry in place of red meat and be sure to remove the skin with its underlying layer of fat.

- **Butter and margarine** contribute about 24 per cent of the fat in the diet. Low-fat spreads can be substituted for these, although their high water content makes them unsuitable for cooking unless you use specially adapted recipes. Eat foods such as bread and crispbread without butter or margarine – if interesting toppings are used, you will not miss them. Say farewell to the knob of butter on vegetables – instead, simply sprinkle with freshly chopped herbs. Jacket potatoes are delicious served with a yogurt dressing rather than butter and go for vegetable-based sauces rather than the fat and flour varieties.

- **Cakes, pastries and biscuits** provide a further 6 per cent of invisible fat in the diet, so it is worth considering eating fruit or scones and sweetened varieties of bread instead and, of course, these alternatives also provide some fibre.

- **Whole milk** provides about 12 per cent of the fat in the diet so use semi-skimmed or skimmed milk instead as the average fat content of these milks is 3.9 per cent, 1.6 per cent and 0.1 per cent respectively.

- **Cheese** contributes about 5 per cent of the fat in the diet so it may be wise to choose some of the lower fat varieties. Edam contains 23 per cent fat and Cheddar 34 per cent; cottage cheese is 1 per cent fat and cream cheese 47 per cent. The range of cheeses with reduced content is worth trying, for example, Cheddar-type.

Also, why not try really strong flavoured cheeses such as 'Extra' mature Cheddar or Parmesan and simply use less to flavour your recipes?
- **Cream** accounts for approximately 2 per cent of the fat in the diet. Try some delicious alternatives such as low-fat yogurt or fromage frais.

In Britain we have a tendency to eat much more fat than is needed. The Department of Health has recommended that the total fat in the diet from food sources (excluding alcohol) should form about 35 per cent of the energy intake. The amount of energy derived from fat is 42 per cent.

Recipe facts

- Whenever possible use wholemeal flour and pasta and brown rice rather than the white varieties.
- Reduce fat – use skimmed or semi-skimmed milk, low-fat yogurt and cheese and choose polyunsaturated margarine.
- Don't add salt during cooking.
- Avoid peeling fruit and vegetables, just wash them thoroughly and, if necessary, peel them thinly with a good peeler rather than a knife.
- Buy canned fruit and vegetables without added sugar or salt.
- Avoid the use of fish canned in oil.
- Follow imperial or metric measures, don't mix the two.
- Unless otherwise stated, use size 3 (medium) eggs.

All recipes are suitable for freezing unless stated otherwise. If you intend to freeze a dish, assemble it in a freezer proof container or transfer it to one.

Savoury protein recipes

Chicken in Tuna Sauce
Chicken with Sweetcorn
Eastern Chicken
Braised Beef and
  Vegetables
Corned Beef Pie
Kidney Yogurt Nests
Pork with Apple
Sweet-and-sour Pork
Crab Salad
Fish Cakes with Chunky
  Tomato Sauce
Fish Crumble
Fish Gratinée
Friday Pie
Hearty Fish Stew
Mackerel Salad
Premium Plaice
Salad Nicoise
Salmon en Papillotes
Smoked Cod Charlotte

Tuna Dip with Crudités
Cheesy Vegetables
Frittata
Macaroni Cheese
Nestled Eggs
Savoury Egg Supper
Spinach Gnocchi with
  Chunky Tomato Sauce
Vegetable Pancakes
  (Crêpes)
Bean Feast
Bean and Mushroom Pâté
Chick Pea (Garbanzo) and
  Tuna Salad
Lentil Pie
Mixed Vegetable Pie
Nutty Cheese Spaghetti
Split Pea Soup
Stuffed Peppers
Tempeh Tagliatelle
Tofu Pitta Pockets

CHICKEN IN TUNA SAUCE

This recipe can be prepared very quickly in a liquidizer (blender). Simply replace the grated onion with a slice of onion and put all the sauce ingredients into the liquidizer (blender) then process until it forms a thick purée.

Serves 4

Metric/Imperial		American
100g/3½oz	canned tuna, well drained	½ cup
150g/5¼oz	natural/plain yogurt	⅔ cup
4 tbs	mayonnaise	4 tbs
½ tsp	anchovy essence	½ tsp
4 tsp	onion, grated	4 tsp
1 tsp	lemon juice	1 tsp
180g/6oz	canned sweetcorn, drained	1 cup
180g/6oz	courgettes/zucchini, diced	1¼ cups
4 tbs	spring onions/scallions, chopped	4 tbs
2	sweet/red peppers	2
300g/10oz	chicken, cooked and diced	2 cups

1. Mash the tuna until it is smooth, then gradually mix in the yogurt, mayonnaise, anchovy essence, grated onion and lemon juice.
2. Mix the sweetcorn with the courgettes (zucchini) and spring onions (scallions).
3. Put the peppers on the rack of a grill (broiler) pan and cook under a high heat, turning occasionally until they are charred and black all over, then plunge them into

Irritable Bowel Syndrome

cold water. When they are cool enough to handle, peel off the black skins, then cut each one in half and remove the seeds. Reserve half of one pepper, cut the remainder into small dice and mix with the vegetables.

4. Spoon the vegetables evenly over the base of a serving dish. Stir the chicken into the tuna sauce and spoon it over the vegetables.

5. Cut the reserved pepper into thin strips and arrange in a lattice pattern over the chicken.

Note to Cooks

Not suitable for freezing.

CHICKEN WITH SWEETCORN

Supermarkets often sell chicken thighs, but, if they are not available, substitute 4 large drumsticks.

Serves 4

Metric/Imperial		American
2 tbs	oil	2 tbs
8	chicken thighs, skin removed	8
1 large	onion, chopped	1 large
2 rashers	lean bacon, rind removed, chopped	2 slices
30g/1oz	wholemeal/wholewheat flour	2 tbs
240ml/8 fl oz	stock	1 cup
1 tbs	tomato purée/tomato paste	1 tbs
340g/12oz	canned sweetcorn, drained	2 cups
1 tbs	chopped tarragon	1 tbs

1. Heat 1 tbs of the oil in a flameproof casserole dish, brown the thighs in the hot oil, adding a little more oil if necessary, then put them on a plate.
2. Add the remaining oil to the casserole dish and stir-fry the onion and bacon for 2–3 minutes.
3. Sprinkle the flour over, stir well, then gradually stir in the stock and tomato purée (tomato paste). Bring to the boil, stirring all the time.
4. Remove the casserole dish from the heat, stir in the sweetcorn, then the chicken and tarragon, cover and cook in a moderate 350°F/180°C/gas mark 4 oven for 1¼–1½ hours until the chicken is tender.

Irritable Bowel Syndrome

EASTERN CHICKEN

You can substitute the basmati rice with brown, easy cook long-grain rice; and start the method at step 2.

Serves 4

Metric/Imperial		American
180g/6oz	brown basmati rice	¾ cup
2 tbs	olive oil	2 tbs
1 small	onion, finely chopped	1 small
1	sweet/red pepper, finely chopped	1
60g/2oz	no-soak dried apricots	⅓ cup
30g/1oz	almonds, unblanched	3 tbs
240ml/8 fl oz	chicken stock	1 cup
4 × 180g/6oz	chicken breasts, partially boned	4

1. Soak the rice in cold water while preparing the other ingredients.
2. Heat the oil in a large saucepan, add the onion and stir-fry for 5 minutes until translucent. Add the red pepper and stir-fry for a further 4 minutes.
3. Stir the apricots, almonds and stock into the saucepan, lay the chicken on top, then cover and simmer for 15 minutes.
4. Remove the chicken from the saucepan, drain the rice and stir into the stock and vegetables. Then lay the chicken back on top of the mixture, cover the saucepan and leave to simmer for 20 minutes.

5. Transfer the chicken to a warm serving plate, but cover the saucepan and continue cooking the rice for 1–2 minutes until fluffy and separate and all the stock has been absorbed. Spoon the rice round the chicken and serve.

Note to Cooks

Not suitable for freezing.

BRAISED BEEF AND VEGETABLES

Whole, large joints of meat may be braised to provide a large number of servings but, for a few people, it is often more convenient to buy one piece of meat and cut it into the number of servings required.

Serves 6

Metric/Imperial		American
2 large	leeks	2 large
720g/1½ lb	mixed root vegetables, e.g., carrots, turnips/turnip roots, parsnips, celeriac	1½ lb
Approx. 840g/1¾ lb	braising steak, e.g. flank, brisket, topside/beef chuck	Approx. 1¾ lb
45g/1½oz	wholemeal/wholewheat flour	3 tbs
1½ tbs	oil	1½ tbs
450ml/¾ pint	warm stock	2 cups
	Fresh bouquet garni	

1. Cut the leeks into thick slices 2.5–4cm (1–1½ in) long. Cut the remaining vegetables into similar-sized chunks.
2. Cut the meat into six pieces and turn in the flour to coat.
3. Heat 1 tbs of the oil in a large flameproof casserole dish (if you don't have one, use a large saucepan, then transfer the vegetables and meat to an ovenproof dish). Turn the meat in the hot oil until it has lightly browned all over, then transfer it to a plate.

4. Add the remaining oil to the dish, then add the leeks and stir-fry for 1–2 minutes. Add the other vegetables and stir-fry for 2–3 minutes.
5. Sprinkle any remaining flour over the vegetables and stir well. Pour the stock into the casserole, add the bouquet garni and lay the meat on top.
6. Tightly cover the casserole and cook at 300°F/150°C/gas mark 2 for 2½ hours, or until the beef is tender.

CORNED BEEF PIE

If you don't have a 1.1 litre (2 pint/5 cup) ovenproof dish, you can use a slightly smaller dish but place it on a baking tray (sheet) just in case it boils over during cooking.

Serves 4

Metric/Imperial		American
720g/1½ lb	potatoes	1½ lb
240g/8oz	leeks, roughly sliced	2 cups
45g/1½oz	margarine	3 tbs
45g/1½oz	wholemeal/wholewheat flour	⅜ cup
300ml/½ pint	milk	1⅓ cups
90g/3oz	hard cheese, finely grated	¾ cup
360g/12oz	corned beef, chopped or mashed	12 slices

1. Cut the potatoes into large chunks and boil for 10 minutes, then add the leeks and cook for a further 8 minutes, or until the potatoes and leeks are just cooked. Drain them well.
2. Melt the margarine in a small saucepan over a moderate heat.
3. Add the flour and cook for 1–2 minutes, stirring all the time.
4. Remove the saucepan from the heat and gradually add the milk. Return to the heat and bring to the boil, stirring all the time. Boil gently for 1–2 minutes until it has thickened.

5. Turn off the heat, sprinkle in about two-thirds of the cheese and stir until the cheese has melted, then add the corned beef.

6. Spoon the cooked potato and leeks into a food processor and process for a few seconds (take care not to process any longer or the potatoes will become 'gluey' in texture).

7. Spoon the cheese and corned beef sauce into an oven-proof dish. Spoon the leek and potato mixture evenly over the top and roughen with a fork. Sprinkle the remaining cheese over the top.

8. Bake at 400°F/200°C/gas mark 6 for about 25 minutes, until the topping is bubbling and golden brown.

KIDNEY YOGURT NESTS

Wholewheat noodles may be used in place of rice.

Serves 2

Metric/Imperial		American
6 large	lamb's kidneys	6 large
90g/3oz	baby corn-on-the-cob	½ cup
1 small	onion	1 small
3–4 tsp	oil	3–4 tsp
120g/4oz	mushrooms	2 cups
15g/½ oz	wholemeal/wholewheat flour	⅛ cup
150ml/5 fl oz	natural/plain yogurt	⅔ cup
120g/4oz	long-grain easy-cook brown rice	½ cup
	parsley to garnish	

1. Remove the outer skin from the kidneys, cut them in half lengthways and cut out the cores. (*Note* You may find it easiest to do this by snipping them with a pair of kitchen scissors.) Cut each kidney into three slices.
2. Cut the corn-on-the-cobs into 12mm (½ in) slices and finely slice the onion, separating each slice into rings.
3. Heat 2 tsp of the oil in a saucepan, add the onion and stir-fry until the rings are limp. Add another tsp of the oil to the pan together with the slices of kidney and stir-fry for 5 minutes.
4. Cut any large mushrooms into thick slices, halve the medium-sized ones and leave very small ones whole,

then add to the pan and keep stirring over a moderate heat until the juices run from them.

5. Cook the rice according to the packaging instructions until the grains are fluffy and separate.

6. Sprinkle the flour over the mushrooms, stir well, add the corn, then gradually add the yogurt. Simmer gently for 12 minutes, stirring occasionally, until the kidneys are just cooked (do not overcook them or they will become rubbery).

7. Divide the rice between 2 warm serving plates, making a ring of rice around the edge of each plate. Then spoon the kidneys and their sauce into the centre and garnish with the chopped parsley.

PORK WITH APPLE

This simple recipe takes only a few minutes to prepare.

Serves 4

Metric/Imperial		*American*
2 × 240g/8oz	cooking apples	2 medium
2 large	onions	2 large
840g/1¾ lb	pork, lean and boned	1¾ lb
3 tbs	redcurrant jelly	3 tbs
240ml/8 fl oz	strong vegetable or chicken stock	1 cup

1. Peel and core the apples, then slice thinly to make apple rings.
2. Thinly slice the onions and separate into rings.
3. If the pork is in one piece, slice it to a thickness of about 2cm (¾ in). Spread the redcurrant jelly thickly over the pork then cut the meat into 5cm (2 in) cubes.
4. Arrange a third of the apple rings in the bottom of a flameproof casserole dish, cover with half the onion rings, then half the pork and repeat these layers, ending with the remaining apple rings.
5. Pour the stock over the pork and apples, cover the dish and bake at 325–350°F/170–180°C/gas mark 3–4 for 1½ hours until the pork is tender.
6. Spoon the pork, apples and onions onto 4 warm serving plates. Put the casserole dish back on the hob and boil the stock fiercely over a high heat for 3 minutes to reduce. Spoon the stock over each portion.

Savoury protein recipes

SWEET-AND-SOUR PORK

Use young, very small mange tout (snowpeas) as these have the best flavour. This recipe is not recommended for freezing as there would be too little sauce to reheat all the ingredients and maintain the crisp texture of the vegetables.

Serves 4

Metric/Imperial		American
480–600g/ 1–1¼ lb	pork loin chops or shoulder steaks/shoulder butt, lean and boned	1–1¼ lb
1 tbs	oil	1 tbs
120g/4oz	mange tout/snowpeas, topped and tailed	1 cup
1 medium	onion, finely chopped	1 medium
1 small	sweet/red pepper, deseeded and chopped	1 small
90g/3oz	canned bamboo shoots, drained	⅔ cup
2 tbs	tomato purée/tomato paste	2 tbs
1 tbs	sugar	1 tbs
1½ tbs	soy/soya sauce	1½ tbs
2½ tbs	vinegar	2½ tbs
6 tbs	water	6 tbs
1½ tbs	wholemeal/wholewheat flour	1½ tbs

1. Lay the pork on the rack of a grill (broiler) pan and cook under moderate heat, turning once, until cooked.
2. While the pork is cooking, heat the oil in a heavy-based saucepan and add the onion. Stir round, then cover tightly and leave over a low heat for 3–4 minutes.
3. Add the red pepper, stir well, then cover tightly and leave for 3–4 minutes.
4. Add the mange tout (snowpeas) and bamboo shoots to the onion and pepper, stir, cover and leave for a further 4–5 minutes.
5. Meanwhile, blend the tomato purée (tomato paste) with the sugar, soy/soya sauce, vinegar and water.
6. Cut the pork into thin strips about 5cm (2 in) long.
7. Sprinkle the flour over the vegetables, stir well, then gradually add the blended sauce and pork. Bring to the boil, stirring all the time, simmer for 3 minutes, then serve.

Note to Cooks

Not suitable for freezing.

CRAB SALAD

This salad makes a refreshing lunch for 2 people. If you wish to serve more people, simply multiply the ingredients as necessary.

Serves 2

Metric/Imperial		American
90g/3oz	wholemeal/wholewheat pasta shapes	¾ cup
90g/3oz	radishes, chopped	9 small
90g/3oz	cucumber, diced	1½ in piece
2	stuffed olives, thinly sliced	2
120g/4oz	white crabmeat, canned and drained or frozen, thawed	3¼ cup
2 tsp	lemon juice	2 tsp
2 tbs	natural/plain yogurt	2 tbs

1. Cook the pasta in boiling water according to the instructions on the packet, then drain well and leave to cool.
2. Mix the cold pasta with the radishes, cucumber, stuffed olives and crabmeat.
3. Stir the lemon juice with the yogurt, pour over the salad and mix well.

Note to Cooks

Not suitable for freezing.

FISH CAKES WITH
CHUNKY TOMATO SAUCE

These fish cakes taste especially good with their home-made tomato sauce. If you prefer, they may be served on their own, but this would decrease the amount of dietary fibre.

Serves 4

Metric/Imperial		*American*
360g/12oz	potato, cooked	1½ cups
360g/12oz	canned salmon or tuna, drained	2 cups
3–4 tbs	chopped chives	3–4 tbs
1 large	egg	1 extra large
3 tbs	milk	3 tbs
15g/½ oz	wholemeal/wholewheat flour	⅛ cup
75g/2½oz	wholemeal/wholewheat breadcrumbs, made from 3 days old bread or fairly dry bread	1¼ cups
	oil for greasing	
½ quantity	Chunky Tomato Sauce (see page 160)	½ quantity

1. Mash the potatoes until smooth, add the fish and chives and mash once again.

2. Beat the egg and milk together, then spoon 3 tbs of it into the fish mixture and mix well. Pour the remainder onto a small plate.

3. Divide the fish mixture into 8 equal amounts, dust the work surface with the flour and, using your hands and a palette knife (narrow spatula) shape each into a round about 2.5cm (1 in) thick.

4. Sprinkle some of the breadcrumbs onto a clean plate. Turn each Fish Cake in the egg and milk then in the breadcrumbs, repeating with the remaining Fish Cakes until all the breadcrumbs have been used up. If some milk and breadcrumbs remain, repeat the process to cover any gaps.

5. Brush a baking tray (baking sheet) with a little of the oil, lay the Fish Cakes on the tray (baking sheet) and bake at 400°F/200°C/gas mark 6 for 25–30 minutes until crisp and beginning to brown.

6. Heat the Chunky Tomato Sauce until steaming. Serve with the hot Fish Cakes.

FISH CRUMBLE

This dish is full of flavour and makes a delicious meal that is especially welcome on a chilly winter's day.

Serves 4

Metric/Imperial		American
180g/6oz	leeks	1 large
180g/6oz	carrots	2 medium
2 large	sticks/stalks celery	2 large
397g/14oz	canned tomatoes	4 cups
1 tsp	chopped basil	1 tsp
1 tbs	chopped parsley	1 tbs
6 tbs	weak stock or water	6 tbs
600g/1¼ lb	smoked cod or haddock fillets, skinned	1¼ lb
1 tbs	cornflour/cornstarch	1 tbs
120g/4oz	wholemeal/wholewheat flour	1 cup
60g/2oz	margarine	¼ cup
60g/2oz	hard cheese, grated	½ cup

1. Cut the leek into 2.5cm (1 in) thick slices. Cut the carrots into large chunks, about 2.5cm (1 in) square. Slice the celery.
2. Put the prepared vegetables, tomatoes, herbs and stock or water in a large saucepan, cover and simmer for 15 minutes.

3. Cut the fish into large pieces, about 5cm (2 in) square. Arrange the fish on top of the vegetables, cover and simmer over a low heat for 10 minutes.

4. Using a slotted spoon, transfer the fish and vegetables to a deep, ovenproof dish.

5. Blend the cornflour (cornstarch) to a smooth paste with about 1 tbs of water, then pour it into the herb and stock or water left in the saucepan. Bring the mixture to the boil, stirring all the time, and boil for 1–2 minutes until it starts to thicken. Spoon about half the sauce over the fish and vegetables and reserve the remainder.

6. Sieve (sift) the flour into a bowl, tip the bran left in the sieve (sifter) back into the flour and, using the tips of your fingers, rub in the margarine until the mixture resembles fresh breadcrumbs. Stir the cheese into the mixture and sprinkle it over the fish and vegetables.

7. Bake at 400°F/200°C/gas mark 6 for 20 minutes. Reheat the reserved sauce and serve it with the Fish Crumble.

FISH GRATINÉE

The spinach and fish sauce is surrounded by a piped border of potatoes, but, if you prefer, the potatoes may be spooned around the edge of the dish then roughened with a fork.

Serves 6

Metric/Imperial		*American*
1kg/2 lb	potatoes	2 lb
500g/1 lb	cod or haddock fillets	1 lb
450ml/¾ pint	milk	2 cups
720g/1½ lb	leaf spinach, frozen	3 cups
45g/1½oz	margarine	3 tbs
45g/1½oz	wholemeal/wholewheat flour	⅜ cup
120g/4oz	hard cheese, grated	1 cup
120g/4oz	peeled prawns	½ cup

1. Cook the potatoes in boiling water, then drain.
2. Lay the cod or haddock in a large saucepan. Reserve 3 tbs of the milk, then pour the remainder into the saucepan, cover and leave over a low heat for about 10 minutes until the fish is just cooked.
3. Mash the potato until smooth, beat in the reserved milk and pipe, using a 2cm (¾ in) fluted nozzle, around the edge of a 25cm (10 in) gratin dish. Place under a grill (broiler) on a *low* heat and complete the recipe.

4. Cook the spinach according to the instructions on the packet, then drain well.

5. Meanwhile drain the cod or haddock, reserve the milk, flake the fish into large pieces, discard the skin and any bones.

6. Melt the margarine in a saucepan, add the flour and cook gently for 1 minute, stirring all the time. Blend the milk into the flour and margarine mixture and bring to the boil, stirring continuously. Stir in three quarters of the cheese, the cooked cod or haddock and the prawns. Stir until the cheese has completely melted.

7. Spoon the spinach into the gratin dish, inside the ring of potato, then spoon the cheese and fish sauce over the spinach and sprinkle the remaining cheese over the top. Then grill (broil) under a moderate heat until golden and bubbling.

FRIDAY PIE

This is an excellent way of using up cooked vegetables. If you prefer, substitute the sweetcorn, peas and carrots with 180g (6oz) mixed vegetables of your choice.

Serves 4

Metric/Imperial		American
720g/1½ lb	potatoes	1½ lb
360ml/12 fl oz	milk	1⅓ cups
450g/1 lb	skinless haddock or cod fillet	1 lb
1–2 slices	onion	1–2 slices
4 tsp	chopped parsley	4 tsp
45g/1½oz	margarine	3 tbs
45g/1½oz	wholemeal/wholewheat flour	⅜ cup
4 tsp	finely chopped chives or spring onions/scallions	4 tsp
60g/2oz	sweetcorn, frozen and cooked or tinned/canned and drained	⅓ cup
60g/2oz	cooked peas	⅓ cup
60g/2oz	cooked carrots	⅓ cup
2	eggs, hard-boiled/hard-cooked and chopped	2
30g/1oz	hard cheese, grated	¼ cup

1. Cook the potatoes in boiling water, then drain and mash well, beating in 3–4 tbs of the milk.

2. Pour the remaining milk into a saucepan, add the fish, onion slices and parsley, cover and simmer gently over a low heat for 6 minutes.

3. Using a slotted spoon, remove the fish from the milk and flake into large pieces onto a plate, removing any bones. Reserve the milk.

4. Melt the margarine in a saucepan, add the flour and stir over a low heat for 1–2 minutes. Remove from the heat and gradually blend in the reserved milk.

5. Return the sauce to the heat and bring to the boil, stirring all the time. Add the chives or spring onions (scallions), cooked vegetables, fish and eggs and boil for 1 minute, stirring continuously.

6. Spoon the fish and vegetable sauce into a 1.4 l (2½ pint/1¼ quart) pie dish. Spread the mashed potato over the top of the fish mixture. Sprinkle the cheese on top.

7. Bake at 400°F/200°C/gas mark 6 for 20–30 minutes until the Pie is golden brown.

HEARTY FISH STEW

Use a firm-fleshed fish for this recipe so the cooked flesh remains in large flakes.

Serves 4

Metric/Imperial		American
2 tbs	olive oil	2 tbs
180g/6oz	onion, sliced	1 cup
1 small	sweet/red pepper, deseeded and cut into 2.5cm (1 in) squares	1 small
90g/3oz	okra, cut into 2.5cm (1 in) lengths	⅔ cup
120g/4oz	baby corn-on-the-cob, cut into 2.5cm (1 in) lengths	⅔ cup
90g/3oz	fennel bulb, roughly chopped	1 cup
397g/14oz	canned, chopped tomatoes	4 cups
180ml/6 fl oz	vegetable or fish stock	⅔ cup
1½ tbs	chopped parsley	1½ tbs
120g/4oz	small, wholewheat pasta shapes	1 cup
720g/1½ lb	white fish e.g., monkfish, boned and skinned	1½ lb

1. Heat the oil in a large saucepan, add the onion and stir-fry for 3–4 minutes.
2. Stir in the sweet/red pepper, okra, baby corn, fennel, tomatoes, stock and parsley. Bring to the boil, cover

and reduce the heat so that the mixture barely simmers. Leave to cook for 25–30 minutes.

3. Stir the pasta into the vegetable mixture, and add a little more stock if necessary.

4. Cut the fish into large pieces about 5 × 7.5cm (2 × 3 in). Carefully stir the fish into the pasta and vegetable mixture, taking care not to break up the chunks. Cover the saucepan and leave over a low heat to simmer for 10–15 minutes, or until the pasta and fish are cooked.

MACKEREL SALAD

The sharp flavour of the plums and lemon juice make a good contrast to the oily fish.

Serves 4

Metric/Imperial		American
360g/12oz	potatoes, cooked	1½ cups
240g/8oz	plums	7 medium
240g/8oz	mackerel, cooked and flaked	1½ cups
4 tbs	lemon juice	4 tbs
4 tbs	natural/plain yogurt	4 tbs

1. Dice the potatoes.
2. Halve the plums, remove the stones (pits) then chop the fruit into small pieces.
3. Mix the mackerel with the diced potatoes and chopped plums
4. Stir the lemon juice and yogurt together then stir into the mackerel mixture.

Note to Cooks

Not suitable for freezing.

PREMIUM PLAICE

Use freshly grated Parmesan cheese – the flavour is far superior to the pre-grated variety.

Serves 2

Metric/Imperial		American
4 × 90g/3oz	plaice fillets	4 medium
30g/1oz	wholemeal/wholewheat flour	2 tbs
1 small	egg, beaten	1 medium
60g/2oz	fresh wholemeal/ wholewheat breadcrumbs	1 cup
30g/1oz	Parmesan cheese, finely grated	¼ cup
4 tsp	oil	4 tsp
240g/8oz	broccoli, separated into florets with 1.25cm/½ in of stalk	2 cups
15g/½ oz	margarine	1 tbs
1 large	banana, peeled	1 large
15g/½ oz	flaked/slivered almonds, toasted	⅛ cup

1. Remove the black skin from the plaice, but leave the white skin.
2. Sprinkle the flour onto one plate, pour the beaten egg onto a second and mix the breadcrumbs and Parmesan cheese together on a third.

3. Turn the plaice fillets in the flour, then the egg and, lastly, the cheese and breadcrumbs, coating them well. (If any egg and breadcrumbs remain once all the fillets have been coated, repeat the procedure, filling in any gaps.)
4. Lay a piece of foil over the rack of a grill (broiler) pan, brush with 1½–2 tsp of the oil. Lay the plaice fillets on the greased foil and drizzle the remaining oil over the top. Cook under a moderate to hot grill (broiler), about 5–7.5cm (2–3 in) away from the heat for 8 minutes, turning once until the plaice is cooked and the breadcrumbs are crisp and golden brown.
5. While the fish is cooking, cook the broccoli in boiling water for 7 minutes, then drain well.
6. Melt the margarine in a saucepan. Slice the banana into 1.25cm (½ in) thick diagonal slices. Turn the banana in the hot margarine. Cook for 1–2 minutes.
7. Add the drained broccoli with the almonds to the banana and stir-fry for 30 to 40 seconds.
8. Serve the plaice with the broccoli, banana and almond mixture immediately.

Note to Cooks

Not suitable for freezing.

SALADE NICOISE

Serve this salad with warm, crusty wholemeal (wholewheat) bread. Assemble all the ingredients just before serving.

Serves 6

Metric/Imperial		*American*
1 tbs	wine vinegar	1 tbs
4 tbs	olive oil	4 tbs
1 tsp	chopped basil	1 tsp
1 tsp	chopped oregano	1 tsp
1 tsp	chopped parsley	1 tsp
Approx. ¼	iceberg/crisphead or cos/romaine lettuce	Approx. ¼
180g/6oz	new potatoes, cooked	¾ cup
120g/4oz	dwarf French/fine green beans, cooked	1 cup
300g/10oz	tomatoes	4 medium
10cm/4 in length	cucumber	4 in length
3 tbs	spring onions/scallions, chopped	3 tbs
200g/7oz	canned tuna, drained	1 cup
2	eggs, hard-boiled/hard-cooked	2
50g/1¾oz	can anchovy fillets, drained	1 small
60g/2oz	black olives	15
	few sprigs of basil or parsley	

1. Whisk (beat) the vinegar with the oil, basil, oregano and parsley to make the dressing.
2. Shred the lettuce into a serving bowl and spoon a little of the dressing evenly over the top.
3. Slice the potatoes and arrange them, overlapping, on top of the lettuce.
4. Arrange the beans over the potato slices.
5. Spoon a little of the dressing over the potatoes and beans.
6. Cut the tomatoes into thin wedges and dice the cucumber, then scatter them and the spring onions (scallions) into the salad bowl. Drizzle half of the remaining dressing over the top.
7. Flake the tuna into large pieces and roughly chop the eggs. Spoon the tuna and eggs on top of the salad.
8. Cut the anchovy fillets in half lengthways and arrange in a lattice pattern over the tuna and eggs. Place the olives decoratively between the anchovy fillets.
9. Spoon the remaining dressing over the Salade Nicoise and garnish with the sprigs of basil or parsley.

Note to Cooks

Not suitable for freezing.

SALMON EN PAPILLOTES

Although we usually recommend polyunsaturated margarine, this recipe is one of the exceptions as unsalted butter adds a delicious, slightly creamy flavour to the salmon.

Serves 2

Metric/Imperial		*American*
30g/1oz	stick/stalk celery, plus its leaves	1 medium
90g/3oz	leek	1 small
90g/3oz	carrot	1 medium
60g/2oz	broccoli florets	½ cup
600ml/1 pint	water	2½ cups
15g/½oz	unsalted butter	1 tbs
2 × 210g/7oz	salmon steaks	2 medium
2 slices	lemon	2 slices
450g/1 lb	potatoes, diced	2⅔ cups
1 small	egg	1 medium

1. Cut the celery, leek, and carrot, into very thin slices. Slice the stems of the small broccoli florets as thinly as possible, and divide the florets into 2.5cm (1 in) lengths.
2. Boil the water in a saucepan, add the celery, cover and boil for 2 minutes. Add the carrot and boil for a further 2 minutes, then add the broccoli stems and florets and boil for 2 more minutes. Drain all the cooked vegetables.

3. Melt the butter in a small saucepan, then add the leeks to the melted butter and stir-fry for 4 minutes until they become limp.

4. Spoon equal amounts of the vegetables onto two 20cm (8 in) square pieces of foil and lay a salmon steak on top of the vegetables. Chop the celery leaves and scatter over the salmon, lay a slice of lemon on top. Fold the foil over the salmon to make 2 neat packages.

5. Put the *papillotes* onto a baking tray (sheet) and bake at 350°F/180°C/gas mark 4 for 20 minutes, or until the salmon is just cooked.

6. Meanwhile, cook the potatoes in boiling water for about 15 minutes until tender, drain them and mash well. Then beat the egg into the potato.

7. Spoon the mashed potato into a piping bag fitted with a 2cm (¾ in) fluted nozzle and pipe the potato around the edge of 2 small gratin dishes. Then brown under a hot grill (broiler).

8. Transfer the salmon and vegetables from the foil to the hot dishes and serve immediately.

Note to Cooks

Not suitable for freezing.

SMOKED COD CHARLOTTE

This recipe makes a substantial meal and only needs a mixed salad or a few mixed vegetables as an accompaniment.

Serves 4

Metric/Imperial		American
75g/2½oz	margarine	5 tbs
45g/1½oz	wholemeal/wholewheat flour	⅜ cup
120g/4oz	canned sweetcorn, drained	⅔ cup
360ml/12 fl oz	milk	1½ cups
600–750g/ 1¼–1½ lb	smoked cod or haddock fillet	1¼–1½ lb
120g/4oz	wholemeal/wholewheat breadcrumbs	2 cups
90g/3oz	hard cheese, grated	¾ cup
3	tomatoes, sliced	3

1. Melt 45g (1½oz or 3 tbs) of the margarine in a saucepan, add the flour and stir over a moderate heat for 1–2 minutes, then remove from the heat.
2. Put the sweetcorn in a liquidizer (blender), add the milk and process for about 30 seconds (a few pieces of sweetcorn will remain: it will not form a smooth purée).
3. Gradually blend the sweetcorn and milk into the margarine and flour.
4. Remove the skin from the fish and cut into 4cm (1½ in) squares.

5. Lightly grease a deep, ovenproof dish (about 17.5cm/7 in in diameter) with half of the remaining margarine, then sprinkle about a third of the breadcrumbs over the base.
6. Return the saucepan with the sweetcorn mixture to the heat and bring to the boil, stirring all the time. Boil for 1–2 minutes, until the sauce has thickened (if the sauce is very thick, add 1–2 tbs more milk). Remove from the heat and stir in the fish and cheese.
7. Spoon half the fish mixture into the dish, spread evenly, then arrange the tomato slices on top. Sprinkle the remaining breadcrumbs over and dot with the remaining margarine.
8. Bake at 400°F/200°C/gas mark 6 for 35–40 minutes until it is bubbling and the breadcrumbs are golden brown.

TUNA DIP WITH CRUDITÉS

Serve this dip as a starter (appetizer). It can be arranged on individual dishes or a large, central plate.

Serves 4

Metric/Imperial		American
For the dip		
100g/3½oz	canned tuna, drained and flaked	½ cup
60g/2oz	curd cheese/ricotta	¼ cup
4 tbs	natural/plain yogurt	4 tbs
1½ tsp	soy/soya sauce	1½ tsp
3	black olives	3
2 tsp	chopped chives or spring onions/scallions	2 tsp
For the crudités		
1 large	stick/stalk celery	1 large
½	sweet/green/bell pepper, deseeded	½
½	sweet/red pepper, deseeded	½
1	courgette/zucchini	1
90g/3oz	carrot	1 medium
60g/2oz	cauliflower florets	½ cup
2 × 45g/1½oz	wholemeal/wholewheat pitta bread	1 large

1. Mash the tuna with the curd cheese (ricotta), yogurt and soy/soya sauce.
2. Remove the stones (pits) from the olives, then chop them finely and stir into the dip, together with the chives or spring onions (scallions). Spoon the dip into a small serving bowl.
3. Cut the celery into 12 sticks 5–7.5cm (2–2½ in) long. Cut each pepper and the courgette (zucchini) into about 8 sticks. Cut the carrot into 12 sticks, about the same length, and separate the cauliflower into small florets.
4. Cut the pitta bread into strips.
5. Arrange the prepared vegetables and pitta strips on a serving plate and serve with the dip.

Note to Cooks

Not suitable for freezing.

CHEESY VEGETABLES

We don't recommend freezing this recipe as it would take so long to cook or reheat that the vegetables would have lost their texture.

Serves 4

Metric/Imperial		American
1 large rasher	lean smoked bacon	1 large slice
1 large	leek, thinly sliced	1 large
180g/6oz	kidney beans, canned or cooked, drained	1 cup
120g/4oz	fennel bulb, chopped	1 cup
90g/3oz	mushrooms	1½ cups
1 tbs	finely chopped basil	1 tbs
1 tsp	tomato purée/tomato paste	1 tsp
3 tbs	water	3 tbs
230g/8oz	canned, chopped tomatoes	1 cup
360g/12oz	potatoes	2 medium
45g/1½oz	margarine	3 tbs
45g/1½oz	wholemeal/wholewheat flour	⅜ cup
360ml/12 fl oz	milk	1½ cups
90g/3oz	hard cheese, grated	¾ cup

1. Remove the rind and all visible fat from the bacon, then grill (broil) it under a moderate heat until cooked but not crisp. Cut it into thin strips across its width.
2. Put the bacon, leek, beans and fennel into a saucepan.

3. Halve or quarter button mushrooms or roughly chop the larger variety. Stir the mushrooms and the basil into the saucepan.

4. Blend the tomato purée (paste) with the water, then stir into the vegetable mixture. Add the chopped tomatoes. Cover the saucepan and cook over a low heat for 12–15 minutes. Remove the saucepan lid and continue cooking, uncovered, for a further 4–5 minutes.

5. Scrub the potatoes thoroughly. Do not peel them. Cook in boiling water for about 10 minutes until they are only just cooked, then drain well. Allow to cool for a few minutes, then cut into thin slices.

6. While the vegetables are cooking, prepare the sauce. Melt the margarine in a small saucepan over a low heat. Add the flour and stir for 1 minute.

7. Gradually blend in the milk and bring to the boil, stirring all the time. Boil for 2 minutes until the sauce is smooth and thick. Remove from the heat and add three quarters of the cheese and stir well until it has melted.

8. Spoon the vegetable mixture into a flameproof dish, arrange the potato slices on top, overlapping them to completely cover the tomato mixture.

9. Spoon the thick cheese sauce over the top. Sprinkle with the remaining cheese and cook under a preheated grill (broiler) until golden brown and bubbling.

Note to Cooks

Not suitable for freezing.

FRITTATA

This is not the traditional Spanish recipe, which would contain more fat to fry the potatoes, but it is very similar as it is cooked slowly until the underside is golden brown, then completed under a hot grill.

Serves 4

Metric/Imperial		American
1½ tbs	oil	1½ tbs
1 medium	onion, finely chopped	1 medium
1	sweet/red pepper, finely chopped	1
60g/2oz	peas, cooked	⅓ cup
120g/4oz	potato, cooked and diced	½ cup
6	eggs, lightly beaten	6
75g/2½oz	hard cheese, grated	heaped ½ cup

1. Heat the oil in a large frying pan (skillet) about 25cm (10 in) diameter.
2. Add the onion and stir-fry over a moderate heat for 2–3 minutes.
3. Add the pepper and stir-fry for 3–4 minutes.
4. Stir the peas and potatoes into the pan and spread evenly across the base.
5. Pour the beaten egg into the pan and lower the heat so the Frittata cooks very slowly. Leave for about 15 minutes when, if you lift one side, you will see that the underside is golden brown and the egg has only just

set on top. Sprinkle with the grated cheese and place under a hot grill (broiler) until the cheese has melted.

6. Slide the Frittata onto a serving plate, cut into 4 wedges and serve.

Note to Cooks

Not suitable for freezing.

MACARONI CHEESE

If you are very short of time, instead of baking this recipe, put the dish under a moderately hot grill (broiler) for a few minutes until the topping is golden brown. Creamed tomatoes, sold in cartons or cans, are puréed tomatoes.

Serves 4

Metric/Imperial		American
180g/6oz	wholemeal/wholewheat macaroni	1½ cups
270g/9oz	frozen, mixed vegetables	1½ cups
60g/2oz	margarine	1¼ cups
60g/2oz	wholemeal/wholewheat flour	½ cup
600ml/1 pint	milk	2½ cups
180g/6oz	mature Cheddar/New York Cheddar, and Parmesan cheese, grated	1½ cups
4–6	spring onions/scallions, chopped	4–6
4 tbs	creamed tomatoes	4 tbs
15g/½ oz	wholemeal/wholewheat breadcrumbs	¼ cup

1. Cook the macaroni according to the instructions on the packet, then drain well.
2. Boil or steam the mixed vegetables, then drain well.

3. Melt the margarine in a saucepan over a low heat, then add the flour and stir for 1–2 minutes. Remove the pan from the heat and gradually blend in the milk.
4. Return the pan to the heat and bring the sauce to the boil stirring all the time. Boil for 1–2 minutes. Add 150–165g (5–5½oz) of the cheese and stir until it has melted. Remove the pan from the heat and stir in the macaroni.
5. Stir the drained and cooked vegetables together with the spring onions (scallions) and tomatoes, then spoon them into a deep, ovenproof dish.
6. Spoon the macaroni and cheese sauce over the vegetables and sprinkle the reserved cheese and breadcrumbs over the top. Bake at 400°F/200°C/gas mark 6 for 20 minutes.

Note to Cooks

Not suitable for freezing.

NESTLED EGGS

This recipe makes a substantial snack when served with baked beans or a mixed salad. If you prefer a very firm egg, similar to a hard-boiled (hard-cooked) egg, increase the cooking time by 5–10 minutes.

Serves 2

Metric/Imperial		*American*
1 × 270–300g/ 9–10oz	potato, as round as possible	1 large
Approx. 2 tbs	milk	Approx. 2 tbs
60g/2oz	hard cheese, finely grated	½ cup
2	eggs	2

1. Scrub the potato well, prick all over with a fork and put in a hot 400°F/200°C/gas mark 6 oven for 1–1¼ hours, or until it is cooked. (If you have the oven at a lower temperature cooking a different recipe the potato may be baked at the same time, but it will just take longer to cook. Increase the heat to cook the eggs.)
2. Cut the potato in half, across its widest part. Carefully scoop out the potato, leaving the skins as shells. Mash the potato until it is smooth. Gradually add the milk and then the cheese.
3. Using a 1.25cm (½ in) fluted nozzle, pipe the potato round the inside edge of the potato skins so the potato is about 1.25cm (½ in) above the shells. Alternatively,

spoon the mashed potato as far round the edge of the shell as possible, then, using a fork, draw it up above the sides.

4. Arrange the potato halves on a baking tray (sheet) (if they do not lie evenly, either lodge them in place or lay in small, ovenproof dishes).

5. Break one egg into each potato half and bake for 20 minutes, or until the eggs are set or cooked to your taste.

Note to Cooks

Not suitable for freezing.

SAVOURY EGG SUPPER

The mild herb and cheese sauce used in this recipe can also be served over vegetables or with white fish, such as cod.

Serves 2

Metric/Imperial		American
300g/10oz	potatoes	2 medium
2	eggs	2
15g/½ oz	margarine	1 tbs
15g/½ oz	wholemeal/wholewheat flour	⅛ cup
150ml/¼ pint	milk	⅔ cup
4 tsp	chopped chervil	4 tsp
2 tsp	chopped chives	2 tsp
415g/14½oz	canned mushy/puréed peas	1⅓ cups
45g/1½oz	hard cheese, grated	⅜ cup
1	tomato, sliced	1

1. Cut the potatoes into chunks and cook in boiling water for 15–20 minutes, then drain well.
2. Put the eggs in a small saucepan, cover with cold water, bring to the boil and simmer for 10 minutes.
3. Melt the margarine in a small saucepan, add the flour and cook over a low heat for 1 minute. Remove the saucepan from the heat and gradually blend in the milk, then stir in the chervil and chives and leave to stand.

4. Heat the mushy peas (puréed peas) then remove them from the heat and mash the peas together with the potatoes.
5. Using a piping bag fitted with a 2cm (¾ in) fluted nozzle, pipe a border of the mixture around the edge of a shallow, flameproof dish and keep it warm while completeing the recipe.
6. Remove the shells from the hot, hard-boiled (hard-cooked) eggs, cut each egg into quarters and lay them in the warm dish inside the piped border.
7. Reheat the sauce, stirring all the time, and boil for 1 minute. Remove from the heat, add two thirds of the cheese and stir well until it has melted.
8. Pour the cheese sauce over the eggs, arrange the tomato slices on top and sprinkle the remaining cheese over the top. Cook under a hot grill (broiler) for 1–2 minutes until the cheese is bubbling and just starting to turn golden brown.

Note to Cooks

Not suitable for freezing.

SPINACH GNOCCHI WITH CHUNKY TOMATO SAUCE

This recipe can be made with fresh or frozen whole leaf spinach. Chopped frozen spinach is not suitable.

Serves 4

Metric/Imperial		American
450g/1 lb fresh or 225g/8oz frozen	leaf spinach	1 lb fresh 1 cup frozen
600ml/1 pint	milk	2½ cups
150g/5oz	wholemeal/wholewheat semolina	1¼ cups
150g/5oz	Cheddar/New York Cheddar and Parmesan cheese, finely grated	1¼ cups
2	eggs, lightly beaten	2
60g/2oz	margarine	¼ cup
½ quantity	Chunky Tomato Sauce (see page 160)	½ quantity

1. Wash fresh spinach well, place in a saucepan without additional water, cover and cook over a low heat for about 5 minutes until it becomes limp. Cook frozen leaf spinach according to the instructions on the packet. Drain the spinach well and leave it until cold.

2. Remove as much water as possible from the spinach by squeezing it very hard, preferably in a clean cloth. Chop the spinach.

3. Pour the milk into a medium-sized saucepan and heat gently until it is steaming.
4. Stir in the semolina and bring to the boil over a low heat, stirring all the time. Boil for about 4 minutes until the mixture is so thick the spoon will stand in it.
5. Add 90g (3oz) cheese to the semolina, beat in the chopped spinach and eggs.
6. Use a quarter of the margarine to grease a baking tray (baking sheet) approximately 30 × 22cm (12 × 9 in).
7. Spoon the semolina and spinach mixture onto the greased tray (baking sheet), smooth it out until it is level and leave until completely cold.
8. Cut the spinach and semolina mixture into 4cm (1½ in) squares and arrange overlapping, in an oven-proof dish.
9. Sprinkle the remaining cheese over the dish and bake at 400°F/200°C/gas mark 6 for 30–35 minutes until bubbling and golden brown.
10. Heat the Chunky Tomato Sauce until it is steaming and serve with the Spinach Gnocchi.

Note to Cooks

Not suitable for freezing.

VEGETABLE PANCAKES (CRÊPES)

This recipe is for 6 people, but if you are cooking for three simply halve the quantities and shorten the cooking time to 35–40 minutes.

Serves 6

Metric/Imperial		American
450g/1 lb	young spinach leaves	1 lb
2 tsp	olive oil	2 tsp
60g/2oz	onion, finely chopped	⅓ cup
450g/1 lb	ricotta cheese	2 cups
2	eggs, lightly beaten	2
60g/2oz	Parmesan cheese, finely grated	½ cup
	Pancakes (Crêpes) (see page 149, makes approximately 12 pancakes (crêpes)	
	Chunky Tomato Sauce (see page 160)	

1. Wash the spinach several times to remove all the grit that collects in the leaves.
2. Shake the excess water from the leaves, place in a saucepan without additional water, cover and cook over a low to moderate heat for about 5 minutes. Drain very well, squeezing out as much moisture as possible.

3. Heat the oil in a saucepan or frying pan (skillet), add the onion and stir-fry for 4–5 minutes until translucent.
4. Chop the spinach, then mix it with the ricotta cheese, eggs and Parmesan cheese.
5. Divide the spinach and ricotta mixture equally between the pancakes (crêpes), then roll them up and place in a large ovenproof dish.
6. Spoon the Chunky Tomato Sauce over the pancakes (crêpes), cover the dish and bake at 375°F/190°C/gas mark 5 for about 50 minutes.

Note to Cooks

Not suitable for freezing.

BEAN FEAST

This simple recipe takes less than 5 minutes to prepare. Use a hard cheese that has a really good flavour.

Serves 4

Metric/Imperial		*American*
5 thick slices	wholemeal/wholewheat bread	5 thick slices
75g/2½oz	hard cheese, finely grated	heaped ½ cup
220g/7¾oz	canned, kidney beans, drained	½ cup
220g/7¾oz	canned butter/lima beans, drained	½ cup
440g/15½oz	canned baked beans	2 cups
2	eggs	2
240ml/8 fl oz	milk	1 cup
	margarine for spreading	

1. Cut 3 of the slices of bread into 4 triangles, then lay them in the bottom of a lightly greased 1.4 l (2½ pint/1¼ quart) pie dish and sprinkle 30g (1oz/¼ cup) of the cheese over the top.
2. Mix the kidney beans and butter (lima) beans with the baked beans.
3. Spoon the bean mixture over the bread and cheese in the pie dish and sprinkle the remaining cheese on top.
4. Thinly spread some margarine over the remaining 2 slices of bread, then cut each slice into 4 triangles. Lay

the triangles – margarine side uppermost – on top of the beans and cheese.

5. Lightly beat the eggs and milk together, then strain them over the bread and leave to stand for 20–30 minutes.

6. Bake at 325°F/170C/gas mark 3 for 1 hour.

Note to Cooks

Not suitable for freezing.

BEAN AND MUSHROOM PÂTÉ

Use mushrooms that have a good flavour for this recipe; cap or chestnut mushrooms give a much better flavour than the button variety.

Serves 4

Metric/Imperial		American
30g/1oz	margarine	2 tbs
90g/3oz	onion, chopped	½ cup
180g/6oz	mushrooms, roughly chopped	2¼ cups
180g/6oz	cannelini beans, dried and cooked or canned and drained	1 cup
2 tsp	mushroom ketchup/catsup	2 tsp

1. Melt half the margarine in a saucepan, add the onion, stir round, then cover and reduce the heat as low as possible. Leave to steam for 5–6 minutes.
2. Add the remaining margarine, then the mushrooms and stir-fry for 1–2 minutes. Cover the saucepan and leave over a low heat for 10 minutes.
3. Put the mushrooms, onion, beans and mushroom ketchup (catsup) into a liquidizer (blender) and process until smooth.
4. Spoon the Bean and Mushroom Pâté into 4 small ramekins, level the surface and then roughen it with the prongs of a fork. Chill.

CHICK PEA (GARBANZO) AND TUNA SALAD

This refreshing salad serves 2 people, but the quantities can easily be increased. If you plan to serve a large number of people it would be more economical to use dried chick peas (garbanzos), as they treble their weight when cooked.

Serves 2

Metric/Imperial		American
240g/8oz	canned chick peas/ garbanzos, drained	1⅓ cups
120g/4oz	canned tuna, drained and flaked	¾ cup
180g/6oz	tomatoes	2 medium
90g/3oz	courgette/zucchini	1 small
1 tbs	lemon juice	1 tbs
1 tbs	olive oil	1 tbs
4 tsp	chives, chopped	4 tsp
2 tsp	basil, chopped	2 tsp

1. Mix the chick peas (garbanzos) with the tuna.
2. Pour boiling water over the tomatoes, leave for 30–40 seconds, then drain and slip off their skins. Cut the tomatoes in half first, then cut each half into 3 wedges.
3. Dice the courgette (zucchini) then stir together with the tomato wedges, the chick peas (garbanzos) and tuna.
4. Whisk the lemon juice with the oil and herbs, then pour the dressing over the salad and mix well.

Note to Cooks
Not suitable for freezing.

LENTIL PIE

This vegetarian version of Shepherd's Pie gives generous, tasty portions that will be enjoyed by vegetarians and non-vegetarians alike.

Serves 4

Metric/Imperial		American
2 tsp	oil	2 tsp
1 large or 2 medium	onions, thinly sliced	1 large or 2 medium
120g/4oz	carrot, diced	1 large
120g/4oz	swede/rutabaga, diced	1 cup
2 large	sticks/stalks celery, chopped	2 large
60g/2oz	mushrooms, chopped	1 cup
2 tbs	tomato purée/tomato paste	2 tbs
150ml/¼ pint	creamed tomatoes	⅔ cup
450ml/¾ pint	water	2 cups
180g/6oz	green lentils	1 cup
90g/3oz	split red lentils	½ cup
720g/1½ lb	potatoes	1½ lb
4 tbs	milk	4 tbs
100g/3½ oz	hard cheese, grated	heaped ¾ cup
2–3 tsp	yeast extract	2–3 tsp

1. Heat the oil in a large saucepan, then add the onions and stir-fry for about 8 minutes until limp and golden.

2. Add the carrot, swede (rutabaga), celery and mush-rooms to the saucepan and stir.

3. Blend the tomato purée (tomato paste) with the creamed tomatoes and water, then stir into the vegetable mixture. Add the lentils. Bring to the boil over a moderate heat then stir well. Reduce the heat, cover the saucepan, and leave to simmer gently for about 50 minutes, stirring occasionally, until the lentils are cooked.

4. While the vegetable mixture is simmering, cook the potatoes in boiling water, then drain and mash with the milk.

5. Beat about three-quarters of the cheese into the mashed potato.

6. Add the yeast extract to the vegetable mixture (this should not be added earlier as the salt in the extract may cause the skins of the lentils to harden).

7. Spoon the lentil mixture into a 1.8 l (3 pint/2½ quart) ovenproof dish. Spread the mashed potato over the top and roughen with the prongs of a fork. Sprinkle the remaining cheese over the mashed potato. Bake at 375°F/190°C/gas mark 5 for 20–30 minutes. The Lentil Pie may be browned under a hot grill (broiler).

MIXED VEGETABLE PIE

This recipe is very versatile. For example, dried, cooked and drained kidney beans may be used in place of some of the tofu.

Serves 4

Metric/Imperial		American
1 small	aubergine/eggplant	1 small
	salt	
1 tbs	oil	1 tbs
1 large	onion, or 2 leeks, chopped	1 large
2	sticks/stalks celery, chopped	2
230g/8oz	canned, chopped tomatoes	2 cups
150ml/¼ pint	stock	⅔ cup
60g/2oz	lentils	⅓ cup
300g/10oz	smoked tofu, diced	1¼ cups
680g/1½ lb	parsnips	1½ lb
210g/7oz	quark	1 cup
2 tsp	margarine	2 tsp

1. Cut the aubergine (eggplant) into chunks, place in a colander or sieve (strainer) and sprinkle liberally with salt. Leave for about 30 minutes to allow the bitter juices to drip away. Rinse well under running cold water and pat dry with kitchen paper (paper towels).
2. Heat the oil in a saucepan, add the onion or leeks and stir-fry for 4 minutes. Add the celery, stir round, reduce the heat, cover and leave to cook gently for 5 minutes.

3. Stir the tomatoes, stock, aubergine (eggplant), lentils and tofu into the saucepan, cover and simmer for 15 minutes.
4. Cut the parsnips into chunks and boil in a separate saucepan for about 15 minutes until cooked, drain and mash with the quark.
5. Spoon the vegetable, lentil and tofu mixture into an ovenproof dish, spoon the parsnip mixture over the top, level and pattern the top with a fork, then dot with the margarine.
6. Bake at 400°F/200°C/gas mark 6 for 20 minutes. If desired, place under a hot grill (broiler) for 1–2 minutes to brown the top.

NUTTY CHEESE SPAGHETTI

Serve this recipe with a crisp, mixed salad.

Serves 4

Metric/Imperial		American
75g/3oz	pecan kernels	⅔ cup
360g/12oz	wholemeal/wholewheat spaghetti	12 ounce
240g/8oz	quark	1 cup
120g/4oz	curd cheese/ricotta	½ cup
120g/4oz	smoked hard cheese, finely grated	1 cup

1. Spread the pecan kernels on a baking tray (baking sheet), put under a moderately hot grill (broiler) and cook until the nuts just begin to brown. Turn the nuts over and continue grilling (broiling) until they are dark brown all over. Leave to cool.
2. Cook the spaghetti according to the instructions on the packet, then drain.
3. Meanwhile, grind the nuts in an electric grinder or mouli grater.
4. Mix the nuts with the quark and curd cheese (ricotta), then spoon the mixture and hot pasta into a pan and stir over a low heat until heated through. Remove from the heat and stir in half the grated cheese.
5. Divide the spaghetti between 4 warm serving plates and sprinkle with the remaining cheese.

SPLIT PEA SOUP

Don't add salt or a salty stock to this soup, as the bacon gives it sufficient flavour. Serve with thick slices of wholemeal (wholewheat) bread.

Serves 4

Metric/Imperial		*American*
180g/6oz	split peas	1 cup
1 tsp	oil	1 tsp
3 rashers	lean bacon, derinded and chopped	3 slices
1 large	onion, finely chopped	1 large
3 or 4	sprigs marjoram	3 or 4
950ml/1¾ pint	stock	4½ cups
1½ tsp	chopped marjoram	1½ tsp

1. Rinse the split peas under running cold water, put in a bowl, cover with double their volume of cold water and leave for about 6 hours or overnight.
2. Heat the oil in a large saucepan, add the bacon, stir round, then add the onion and stir-fry for 4–5 minutes.
3. Drain the split peas and transfer to the saucepan; add the sprigs of marjoram and stock. Bring to the boil, stir well, cover and reduce the heat as low as possible. Simmer for 1¾–2 hours.
4. Ladle the soup into four warm soup bowls and sprinkle with the chopped marjoram.

STUFFED PEPPERS

Use a strong-flavoured cheese such as mature Cheddar.

Serves 4

Metric/Imperial		American
180g/6oz	wholemeal/wholewheat bread, crusts removed	5 large slices
180g/6oz	cashew nuts/kernels	1½ cups
180g/6oz	hard cheese, finely grated	1½ cups
2 tsp	tomato purée/tomato paste	2 tsp
450g/1 lb	tomatoes	1 lb
4 tsp	chopped chives	4 tsp
1 tsp	chopped oregano	1 tsp
4 large	sweet/red peppers	4 large

1. Put a slice of bread in a liquidizer (blender) and process to form breadcrumbs, put to one side.
2. Put the remaining bread and the cashew nuts into the liquidizer (blender) and process to form crumbs, tip into a bowl.
3. Reserve about 30g (1oz/¼ cup) of the cheese. Mix the remainder with the nut and bread mixture, then add the tomato purée (tomato paste).
4. Cover the tomatoes with boiling water, leave for 40 seconds, then drain and slip off their skins.
5. Chop the tomatoes into small pieces then add to the bread, nut and cheese mixture, together with the herbs.

6. Cut the peppers in half lengthways, remove all the seeds, then boil a large saucepan of water for 3 minutes. Drain well.
7. Pat the inside of the peppers with kitchen paper (paper towels), then divide the bread mixture between the pepper halves, level the surface and sprinkle the reserved cheese and breadcrumbs over the top.
8. Put the peppers in a lightly greased ovenproof dish and bake at 375°F/190°C/gas mark 5 for 30–35 minutes until the peppers are cooked and the topping golden.

Note to Cooks

Not suitable for freezing.

TEMPEH TAGLIATELLE

Tempeh is sold frozen in blocks. Leave it to thaw before incorporating in recipes. Unlike tofu, tempeh requires cooking before it is eaten.

Serves 6

Metric/Imperial		American
2 tbs	olive oil	2 tbs
360g/12oz	onion, thinly sliced	2 cups
1 large	sweet/red pepper, deseeded and diced	1 large
1 large	bell/green pepper, deseeded and diced	1 large
2 × 397g/14oz	cans chopped tomatoes	6 cups
2 tbs	tomato purée/tomato paste	2 tbs
240ml/8 fl oz	vegetable stock	1 cup
1–2 tbs	finely chopped oregano	1–2 tbs
2 tbs	soy/soya sauce	2 tbs
2 × 240g/8oz blocks	tempeh, thawed and diced	1 lb
360g/12oz	wholewheat tagliatelle	3 cups

1. Heat the oil in a large saucepan, add the onion and stir-fry for 5 minutes until the slices are limp and translucent.
2. Add the red and green peppers and stir-fry for a further 3–4 minutes.
3. Add the tomatoes, tomato purée (tomato paste), stock oregano and soy/soya sauce to the vegetables and

bring to the boil, stirring all the time. Reduce the heat, cover and leave to simmer gently for 30 minutes, stirring occasionally.

4. Add the tempeh to the pan and leave to simmer for a further 10 minutes.

5. Meanwhile, cook the tagliatelle in boiling water according to the instructions on the packet.

6. Drain the tagliatelle and serve it on 6 plates with the vegetable and tempeh sauce spooned over the top.

TOFU PITTA POCKETS

These moist burgers may be served as the protein component of a main meal. If so, allow two burgers per person.

Serves 6

Metric/Imperial		American
300g/10oz	firm tofu	1¼ cups
110g/3½oz	wholemeal/wholewheat flour	⅞ cup
5 tbs	tomato purée/tomato paste	5 tbs
3 tbs	grated onion	3 tbs
4 tbs	soy/soya sauce	4 tbs
	oil for greasing	
6 × 75g/2½oz	wholemeal/wholewheat pitta breads	6 medium
	a few lettuce leaves, shredded	
180g/6oz	tomatoes, sliced	2
	a few onion rings	

1. Grate, or chop, the tofu into a bowl. Reserve 1 tablespoon of flour and combine the remainder with the tofu, tomato purée (tomato paste), onion and soy/soya sauce and mix them together well.
2. Divide the tofu mixture into 6 balls.
3. Sprinkle the work surface with a little of the reserved flour and, using a palette knife (narrow spatula), shape each ball into a flat burger, about 1.25cm (½in) thick, adding more of the flour as necessary.

4. Lay a piece of foil in the grill (broiler) pan and brush a little oil over the foil. Lay the burgers on the foil and brush them with a little oil. Grill (broil) under a very hot preheated grill (broiler) for about 3 minutes. Using the palette knife (narrow spatula), carefully turn the burgers over, brush with a little more oil and cook for 3 minutes.

5. Warm the pitta breads, split each one in half width-ways and spread out a little of the lettuce evenly in each half. Cut the burgers in half and place one half in each pitta pocket. Arrange the slices of tomato and the onion rings on top of the burgers, close up the pitta breads and serve.

6

Cereal recipes

Breakfast Cereals
Breakfast Crunch
De Luxe Muesli
Economical Muesli
Traditional Scottish
   Porridge

Breads and Scones
'Short Time' Wholemeal
   (Wholewheat) Bread
Soda Bread
Savoury Bread Rolls
Fruity Griddle Scones
Traditional Scones
Tattie Scones
Baguette Sandwich
Bread and Cheese Bake
French Bread Pizza
Rolled Sandwich
Toasted Sandwich

Accompaniments
Bulgar Salad

Rice Salad
Savoury Rice
Savoury Rice Pudding
Melba Toast
Yorkshire Pudding

Tea-time (Afternoon) Favourites
Banana Teabread
Carrot Buns
Date Cake
Sticky Fruit Buns
Eggless Fruit Cake
Yeast Cake
Simple Malt Loaf
Wholesome Carrot Cake

Desserts
Apricot Semolina
Bread Pudding
Fruit and Bread Bake
Fruity Bread Pudding
Pancakes (Crêpes)

BREAKFAST CRUNCH

This recipe may be eaten as a breakfast cereal or used as a topping for desserts.

Serves 10–12

Metric/Imperial		American
180g/6oz	jumbo oats	1¾ cups
180g/6oz	barley flakes	1¾ cups
30g/1oz	wheatgerm	¼ cup
30g/1oz	sesame seeds	3½ tbs
30g/1oz	hazelnut kernels	¼ cup
6 tbs	clear honey	6 tbs
75g/2½oz	margarine	5 tbs

1. Mix the jumbo oats with the barley flakes, wheatgerm and sesame seeds in a bowl.
2. Chop the hazelnuts and add them to the bowl of cereals.
3. Heat the honey and margarine in a saucepan over a low heat and, when the margarine has melted and combined with the honey, pour the mixture into the bowl and stir thoroughly to coat all the ingredients.
4. Spoon the mixture onto a large baking tray (baking sheet) and spread as evenly and thinly as possible.
5. Bake at 375°F/190°C/gas mark 5 for about 30 minutes, stirring every 10 minutes so that the cereal, which browns more quickly round the edge of the baking tray (sheet), is replaced with the lighter cereal from the centre. Cook until all the cereal is golden brown. Leave until completely cold, transfer it to an airtight container.
6. Serve about 45g (1½oz/⅓ cup) as a single serving for breakfast.

Cereal recipes

DE LUXE MUESLI

This muesli is a real treat! If you are unable to find dried papaya or pineapple, just increase the proportions of the other dried fruits.

Serves 10–12

Metric/Imperial		American
180g/6oz	porridge oats	1½ cups
45g/1½oz	wheatgerm	⅜ cup
30g/1oz	barley flakes	⅓ cup
30g/1oz	wheat flakes	⅓ cup
30g/1oz	rye flakes	⅓ cup
30g/1oz	roasted buckwheat/kasha	2 tbs
30g/1oz	mixture of brazil and hazel kernels, roughly chopped	3 tbs
60g/2oz	dried papaya and pineapple, diced	⅜ cup
90g/3oz	dried apricots, peaches and apples, finely chopped	⅔ cup

To serve each portion of muesli:

45g/1½oz	muesli base	⅓ cup
5 tbs	orange juice	5 tbs
2 tbs	natural/plain yogurt	2 tbs
2–3	banana chips (optional)	2–3

1. Mix the porridge oats with the wheatgerm, barley, wheat and rye flakes and buckwheat (kasha) in a bowl.

2. Stir the nuts, dried papaya and pineapple into the cereal mixture.
3. Add the remaining dried fruits to the cereal mixture and stir. Store the muesli in an airtight container.
4. For each portion of De Luxe Muesli, put 45g (1½oz/⅓cup) of the muesli into a cereal bowl. Stir the orange juice into the muesli and keep the bowl in the refrigerator overnight. In the morning, stir the yogurt into the soaked muesli, crush the banana chips and sprinkle over the top. (If preferred, you can omit soaking the muesli overnight.)

ECONOMICAL MUESLI

This low-cost muesli takes only a few minutes to prepare and can be stored for several weeks in an airtight container.

Serves 6–8

Metric/Imperial		American
240g/8oz	porridge oats	2 cups
30g/1oz	wheatgerm	¼ cup
60g/2oz	sultanas/golden seedless raisins	⅓ cup
30g/1oz	walnuts/English walnuts, coarsely chopped	3 tbs

To serve each portion of muesli:

45g/1½oz	muesli base	⅓ cup
4 tbs	milk	4 tbs
140g/5oz	dessert/sweet apple	1 small
1 tbs	yogurt (optional)	1 tbs

1. Mix the porridge oats together with the wheatgerm, sultanas (golden seedless raisins) and walnuts (English walnuts). Store the muesli in an airtight container.
2. For each portion of Economical Muesli, put 45g (1½oz/⅓ cup) of the muesli into a cereal bowl. Add the milk, stir and put the bowl in the refrigerator overnight. In the morning, core and chop the apple. Stir the apple and yogurt into the soaked muesli. (If preferred, you can omit soaking the muesli overnight.)

TRADITIONAL SCOTTISH PORRIDGE

There are many breakfast cereals sold today and several of them are promoted as high fibre. However, the traditional warming dish of porridge makes an excellent start to the day and provides an acceptable amount of fibre. This recipe is made from medium oatmeal and, if you wish to make an authentic porridge, stir it with a spurtle! (A spurtle is a stick shaped like a thistle.)

Serves 1

Metric/Imperial		American
30g/1oz	medium oatmeal	¼ cup
300ml/½ pint	water, or milk and water	1⅓ cups
	salt	

1. Put the oatmeal in a small saucepan. Stir in the milk, or milk and water.
2. Over a moderate heat, bring to the boil, then reduce the heat and simmer gently for 20 minutes, stirring occasionally to prevent it sticking.
3. Stir a little salt into the cooked porridge and spoon into a warm bowl. Serve it on its own or with a little milk and honey or sugar.

'SHORT TIME' WHOLEMEAL (WHOLEWHEAT) BREAD

Adding the 25mg vitamin C tablet means that the bread only needs one rising to produce the texture of traditional home-made bread. If you prefer, you can use dried yeast instead of fresh. Simply follow the manufacturer's directions as to the quantity and, unless otherwise stated, dissolve ½ teaspoon sugar in the warm milk and leave for 10 to 15 minutes until the mixture is frothy, then continue from step 2.

Makes 2 small loaves or 18 rolls

Metric/Imperial		*American*
20g/¾ oz	fresh yeast	scant 2 tbs
Approx	warm milk	1½ cups
450ml/¾ pint	(hand hot, not boiling)	
700g/1½ lb	wholemeal/wholewheat flour	6 cups
1 tbs	salt	1 tbs
30g/1oz	margarine	2 tbs
25mg	vitamin C tablet	25mg
	extra flour for dusting	

1. Crumble the yeast into a jug, then gradually blend in the warm water.
2. Sieve (sift) the flour and salt into a bowl, tipping the bran remaining in the sieve (sifter) back into the bowl.
3. Rub (cut) in the margarine.
4. Crush the vitamin C tablet into the yeast mixture and stir well until it has dissolved.

5. Make a well in the flour and pour the yeast liquid into it, then mix gently until you have a soft dough. Mix a little longer until the dough leaves the sides of the bowl.

6. Transfer the dough to a lightly floured work surface and knead well, drawing about one-third of the dough up with your fingers and folding it back onto the remaining two-thirds, then pressing it down with the palms of your hands in a rhythmic motion. Stretch the dough and continue kneading for about 10 more minutes until it is smooth.

7. Lightly grease 2 small loaf tins (pans) or 2 baking trays (sheets).

8. If using loaf tins (pans), divide the dough in half, roll each half into rectangles and press them into the loaf tins (pans). If making rolls, divide the dough into a total of 18 pieces and work each into a round or finger shape then put them a little distance apart from each other on the baking trays (baking sheets).

9. Cover the loaves or rolls with a lightly greased piece of polythene and leave somewhere warm (like an airing cupboard) until they are well risen and have doubled in size.

10. Remove the polythene, dust the loaves or rolls with flour and bake in a very hot 450°F/230°C/gas mark 8 oven for about 15 minutes for the rolls, 35–40 minutes for the loaves. Test that the rolls and loaves are cooked by tapping the bottom – they should sound hollow. Transfer the cooked bread to a wire rack and leave to cool.

Cereal recipes

SODA BREAD

This loaf is best eaten very fresh – if possible, while still warm. It can be frozen immediately after it has been cooked and cooled, but should be eaten immediately it has thawed as the texture quickly becomes dry.

Makes 1 small loaf

Metric/Imperial		*American*
360g/12oz	wholemeal/wholewheat flour	3 cups
½ tsp	salt	½ tsp
1½ tsp	bicarbonate of soda/ baking soda	1½ tsp
just under 300ml/½ pint	buttermilk	1¼ cups

1. Sieve (sift) the flour, salt and bicarbonate of soda (baking soda) into a bowl. Tip the bran remaining in the sieve (sifter) back into the bowl.
2. Reserve a tablespoon of buttermilk. Mix the remainder into the dry ingredients with a fork until the mixture forms a soft dough (if it is too dry, add a little more buttermilk).
3. Transfer the dough to a lightly floured work surface and knead it gently until smooth.
4. Put the dough on a lightly greased baking tray (baking sheet) and roll then pat into a circle 2.5–4cm (1–1½ in) thick.

5. Using a sharp knife, score the top of the dough into quarters.
6. Bake in a hot 425°F/220°C/gas mark 7 oven for 20–25 minutes.
7. Transfer the loaf to a cooling rack and leave until it is just warm or cold before serving.

SAVOURY BREAD ROLLS

Fresh yeast is often sold in bread shops, but if you are unable to buy it or prefer to substitute dried yeast, just follow the manufacturer's directions as to the right quantity to use. Unless otherwise stated, dissolve ½ teaspoon sugar in the warm milk and yeast, and leave for 10–15 minutes until the mixture is frothy, then mix it into the flour and continue from step 2.

Serves 10

Metric/Imperial		American
15g/½ oz	fresh yeast	1¼ tbs
Approx. 210ml/7 fl oz	warm milk (hand hot, not boiling)	¾ cup
360g/12oz	wholemeal/wholewheat flour	3 cups
1 tsp	salt	1 tsp
30g/1oz	margarine	2 tbs
75g/2½oz	hard cheese, finely grated	heaped ½ cup
2 tsp	finely grated onion	2 tsp

1. Crumble the yeast into a jug, then gradually blend in the warm milk.
2. Sieve (sift) the flour and salt into a bowl. Tip the bran remaining in the sieve (sifter) into the bowl.
3. Rub (cut) in the margarine.
4. Mix the yeast liquid into the flour until it forms a soft dough.
5. Transfer the dough to a lightly floured work surface

and knead by drawing about one-third of the dough up with your knuckles then press down onto the remaining two-thirds and press with the palms of your hands in a rhythmic action. Knead for about 10 minutes until the dough is smooth and elastic. (Alternatively, mix the dough in a food processor or an electric mixer fitted with a dough attachment for about 3 minutes.)

6. Put the dough in a clean bowl, cover with a piece of lightly greased polythene and leave in a warm place until it has doubled in size (about 1 hour).

7. Return the dough to the lightly floured work surface and press it out to form a square about 22.5cm (9 in) in size. Sprinkle 60g (2oz/½ cup) of the cheese and all the onion evenly over the dough. Fold the corners of the dough into the centre, then knead the dough well for 4–5 minutes.

8. Divide the dough in 10 equal pieces and shape into rolls.

9. Lightly grease 2 baking trays (baking sheets), put 5 rolls on each one, then cover with lightly greased polythene. Leave the rolls in a warm place for about 40 minutes until well risen.

10. Bake the rolls in a very hot 450°F/230°C/gas mark 8 oven for about 15 minutes. Check that the rolls are cooked by gently tapping the base – they should sound hollow.

11. Turn the oven off, arrange the rolls close together, sprinkle with the remaining cheese, return to the oven and leave for 2–3 minutes, until the cheese has begun to melt. Transfer the rolls to a wire rack to cool.

FRUITY GRIDDLE SCONES

Serve these scones warm, halved and spread thinly with butter or margarine.

Serves 3

Metric/Imperial		American
180g/6oz	self-raising wholemeal/ self-rising wholewheat flour	1½ cups
1 tsp	baking powder	1 tsp
30g/1oz	margarine	2 tbs
15g/½ oz	caster/superfine sugar	1 tbs
60g/2oz	dried mixed fruit	⅓ cup
1	egg, beaten	1
Approx. 1 tbs	milk	Approx. 1 tbs
	oil for cooking	

1. Reserve 2 tablespoons flour then sieve (sift) the remainder with the baking powder into a bowl. Tip the bran remaining in the sieve (sifter) into the bowl.
2. Rub (cut) the margarine into the flour until the mixture resembles fresh breadcrumbs.
3. Stir in the caster (superfine) sugar and dried fruit.
4. Gently and gradually, mix the egg and 1 tbs of the milk into the dry ingredients to form a soft, but not sticky, dough.
5. Dust the work surface and a rolling pin with the reserved flour, then roll out the dough on the floured surface to form a rectangle about 1.25–2cm (½–¾ in) thick. Cut it into 6 triangles.

Irritable Bowel Syndrome

6. Heat a griddle or heavy-based frying pan (skillet). When it is hot, add sufficient oil to thinly coat the surface, then lay the scones on top and cook over a moderate heat for 12 minutes, turning once, until golden.

TRADITIONAL SCONES

The combination of white and wholemeal (wholewheat) flours retains the light texture of traditional white scones, but adds a great deal of flavour due to the wholemeal (wholewheat). To make plain scones, omit the dried fruit.

Serves 10

Metric/Imperial		American
120g/4oz	plain/all-purpose white flour	1 cup
120g/4oz	wholemeal/wholewheat flour	1 cup
2½ tsp	baking powder	2½ tsp
45g/1½oz	margarine	3 tbs
1 tbs	soft brown sugar	1 tbs
60g/2oz	dried mixed fruit	⅓ cup
1	egg, lightly beaten	1
Approx. 4 tbs	milk	¼ cup

1. Sieve (sift) the flours and baking powder into a bowl. Tip the bran remaining in the sieve (sifter) into the bowl.
2. Using the tips of your fingers, rub the margarine into the flour until the mixture resembles fresh bread-crumbs.
3. Stir in the sugar and dried fruit.
4. Make a well in the centre of the mixture and pour in the egg and 3 tbs of the milk.

5. Using a round-bladed knife and adding a little more milk if necessary, mix to form a soft, but not sticky, dough.
6. Very lightly knead the dough until smooth.
7. Lightly flour a work surface and roll the dough out until it is about 2cm (¾ in) thick (do not stretch the dough or roll it out any thinner).
8. Cut the dough into rounds using a 5cm (2 in) cutter (cookie cutter). (If it begins to stick, dip it in a little flour then continue.) Lightly knead the trimmings together, re-roll, then cut into more scones. Leave the scones on the work surface for 10–15 minutes.
9. Meanwhile, put a baking tray (baking sheet) in the oven and heat to 450°F/230°C/gas mark 8.
10. Lay a sheet of non-stick baking paper (baking parchment) onto the hot baking tray (baking sheet), then put the scones on top, leaving a little space between them, and bake for 8–10 minutes until they are well risen and golden brown. Then leave them to cool on a wire rack and serve when either still a little warm or cold.

TATTIE SCONES

Although potatoes are the main ingredient, this recipe is included here as scones are often a substitute for bread or cakes.

Serves 4

Metric/Imperial		*American*
450g/1 lb	potatoes	1 lb
30g/1oz	margarine	2 tbs
1 tsp	salt	1 tsp
120g/4oz	self-raising wholemeal/	1 cup
	self-rising wholewheat flour	
	oil for cooking	

1. Peel the potatoes, cut them into chunks and cook in boiling water for 15–20 minutes. Drain them and, while hot, mash with the margarine and salt.
2. Reserve 2–3 tablespoons flour. Mix the remainder into the potatoes to form a soft dough.
3. Sprinkle the reserved flour over a work surface and rolling pin and roll out the dough until it is about 1.25cm (½ in) thick. Cut it into 7.5cm (3 in) triangles.
4. Heat a little oil in a heavy-based griddle or frying pan (skillet) – add only sufficient oil to coat the surface to stop the scones sticking. Lay the scones on the hot surface and cook over a moderate heat for 2–3 minutes until golden, then turn them over and cook the other side. Keep the cooked scones warm while re-rolling the dough, and cooking the remaining mixture.

Note to Cooks

Not suitable for freezing.

Irritable Bowel Syndrome

BAGUETTE SANDWICH

Baguette Sandwiches make quick, appetizing snacks. They also make easily transportable meals – just cover them in foil or clingfilm (saran wrap).

Serves 2

Metric/Imperial		American
1	wholemeal/wholewheat baguette	1
½	or French stick	½
2	eggs, hard-boiled/ hard-cooked	2
227g/8oz	cottage/pot cheese with onion and red pepper, or favourite flavour, or plain/natural	1 cup
2–3 tsp	low-calorie mayonnaise	2–3 tsp
2–3	crisp lettuce leaves	2–3

1. Make a horizontal cut almost, but not completely, through the bread so it remains in one piece.
2. Pull the soft bread out from each half, leaving a little attached to the crusts, and put it into a liquidizer (blender) and process to form breadcrumbs.
3. Shell and mash the hard-boiled (hard-cooked) eggs in a bowl, mix in the breadcrumbs, and cottage (pot) cheese. Stir 2 tsp mayonnaise into the mixture adding a little more to taste if desired.

4. Shred the lettuce leaves and arrange evenly along the bottom half of the bread. Spoon the egg mixture on top of the lettuce, piling it up a little in the centre.
5. Cover with the top half of the bread, cut the baguette in half and serve.

Note to Cooks

Not suitable for freezing.

BREAD AND CHEESE BAKE

This recipe makes a substantial lunch or supper. A crisp mixed salad is the perfect accompaniment.

Serves 4

Metric/Imperial		*American*
180g/6oz	wholemeal/wholewheat bread slices	6
4 tsp	grated onion	4 tsp
120g/4oz	hard cheese, grated	1 cup
450ml/¾ pint	milk	2 cups
3	eggs, lightly beaten	3

1. Cut the bread into 2.5cm (1 in) strips.
2. Arrange a third of the bread evenly over the base of a lightly greased 1.4 l (2½ pint/1½ quart) ovenproof dish.
3. Sprinkle half of the grated onion and a third of the cheese over the bread. Repeat these layers, then arrange the remaining bread and cheese on top.
4. Heat the milk until steaming, then turn off the heat and whisk (beat) in the eggs.
5. Strain the milk and eggs mixture over the layered bread and leave to stand for 15–20 minutes.
6. Cook the Bread and Cheese Bake at 350°F/180°C/ gas mark 4 for 35–40 minutes until just set.

Note to Cooks

Not suitable for freezing.

FRENCH BREAD PIZZA

These bread pizzas are simple to make and yet provide a substantial snack.

Serves 2

Metric/Imperial		American
2 × 12.5cm (5 in) lengths	wholemeal/wholewheat French bread	2 × 5 in lengths
4 tsp	olive oil	4 tsp
1	onion, thinly sliced and separated into rings	1
2 rashers	lean bacon	2 slices
4 tsp	tomato purée/tomato paste	4 tsp
	marjoram or oregano leaves, chopped	
120g/4oz	Mozzarella cheese	½ cup

1. Cut the French bread in half lengthways.
2. Heat the oil in a saucepan, add the onion and stir-fry for 5–6 minutes until the onion rings are limp and golden.
3. Derind the bacon and cook under a moderate grill (broiler). Leave to cool, then cut the bacon into thin strips across the width.
4. Grill (broil) the rounded side of the French bread, then turn and grill (broil) the cut side until it just begins to brown.
5. Spread each piece of bread with tomato purée (tomato paste), scatter the chopped herbs over it and spoon the onion rings evenly on top. Arrange the pieces of bacon on top of the onion.

6. Cut the Mozzarella into 8 slices and lay 2 on top of each pizza.
7. Cook for about 3 minutes under a moderately hot grill (broiler) until the cheese is bubbling and beginning to turn brown.

Note to Cooks

Not suitable for freezing.

ROLLED SANDWICH

These sandwiches can be eaten whole as a substitute for traditional sandwiches or thinly sliced and served as a cocktail snack or an appetizer.

Serves 3

Metric/Imperial		*American*
1 small	wholemeal/wholewheat loaf, 1–2 days old, uncut	1 small
100g/3½oz	canned tuna, well drained	1 cup
60g/2oz	curd cheese/ricotta	¼ cup
1 tbs	natural/plain yogurt	1 tbs
½ tsp	tomato purée/tomato paste	½ tsp
2 tbs	finely chopped sweet/red pepper	2 tbs
1 tbs	finely chopped spring onions/scallions	1 tbs
	lemon juice	

1. Cut the loaf lengthways just above the base to remove the crust.
2. Place the loaf on its side and cut 6 slices along its *length*. Trim all the crusts from the slices, which should give you 6 slices approximately 18 × 7.5cm (6½ × 3 in).
3. Mash the tuna with the curd cheese (ricotta), yogurt, tomato purée (tomato paste), red pepper and spring onions (scallions). Add lemon juice to taste.

4. Spread equal amounts of the tuna mixture over each slice of bread, then roll each one up Swiss-roll (jelly-roll) fashion, rolling from one of the shorter sides to the other.
5. Lay each Rolled Sandwich on a piece of clingfilm (saran wrap) and wrap the roll tightly. Chill for about 3 hours.
6. Remove the clingfilm (saran wrap) from each sandwich and either serve whole or slice thinly and arrange on a serving plate.

Note to Cooks

Not suitable for freezing.

TOASTED SANDWICH

A toasted sandwich makes a quick, appetizing snack. If time allows make a simple salad as an accompaniment. Cook under a grill (broiler) or in an electric sandwich toaster.

Serves 1

Metric/Imperial		American
2 slices	wholemeal/wholewheat bread	2 slices
45g/1½oz	hard cheese, grated or thinly sliced	⅜ cup
30g/1oz slice	corned beef	1 slice
1 small	tomato	1 small
	margarine (optional)	

1. Sprinkle half the cheese on 1 slice of bread.
2. Lay the corned beef on top of the cheese.
3. Slice the tomato and arrange on top of the corned beef.
4. Sprinkle the rest of the cheese over the tomato and top with the second slice of bread.
5. Either grill (broil) the sandwich under a moderate grill (broiler) until golden brown, or thinly spread the outside of the sandwich with margarine and cook in an electric sandwich toaster.

Note to Cooks

Not suitable for freezing.

BULGAR SALAD

Bulgar wheat is cracked wheat that has been partially cooked. It can be found in many supermarkets and health food shops.

Serves 4

Metric/Imperial		American
120g/4oz	bulgar wheat	⅔ cup
1	sweet/yellow or red pepper	1
4	radishes, chopped	4
2 tbs	finely chopped spring onions/scallions	2 tbs
2tbs	olive oil	2 tbs
4 tbs	lemon juice	4 tbs
2 tbs	finely chopped mint leaves (not stems/stalks)	2 tbs

1. Rinse the bulgar wheat under cold running water, drain and put it into a bowl. Cover the bulgar wheat with twice its volume of boiling water and leave until cold.
2. Lay the pepper on the rack of a grill (broiler) pan and cook under a high heat, turning occasionally until it is charred. Put the charred pepper in a bowl of cold water and leave it for a few minutes until cool enough to handle, pull off the charred skin, remove the core and seeds and chop the flesh.
3. Spoon the bulgar wheat into a clean cloth and squeeze hard to remove as much excess water as possible.

Cereal recipes

4. Mix the bulgar wheat with the pepper, radish and spring onions (scallions).
5. Mix the olive oil with the lemon juice and mint and pour this dressing over the bulgar wheat mixture, stirring it well to coat all the ingredients.

Note to Cooks

Not suitable for freezing.

RICE SALAD

Use this as a basic recipe, apples, mandarins, courgettes and mushrooms may also be added as you like.

Serves 4

Metric/Imperial		American
180g/6oz	brown basmati rice	¾ cup
30g/1oz	hazelnut kernels	¼ cup
120g/4oz	pineapple, fresh or canned, drained and diced	¾ cup
30g/1oz	raisins	⅛ cup
½	sweet/red pepper, deseeded and diced	½ medium
½	bell/green pepper, deseeded and diced	½ medium
2–3 tsp	chopped chives	2–3 tsp

1. Soak and cook the rice according to the directions on the packet until the grains are fluffy and separate, then leave to cool.
2. Meanwhile, put the hazelnut kernels into a grill (broiler) pan and cook them under moderate heat until they are golden brown, then roughly chop them and place in a bowl.
3. Stir the pineapple together with the raisins and nuts.
4. Stir the diced peppers, chives and cold rice into the fruit and nut mixture and mix all the ingredients together well, then spoon the Rice Salad into a serving dish.

Note to Cooks
Not suitable for freezing.

SAVOURY RICE

The amount of stock required in this recipe will vary according to the rice and the amount of moisture rendered by the frozen peas. To make sure you have the right level of moisture, cook the dish over a low heat and check that there is sufficient liquid a few minutes before the end of the cooking time.

Serves 4

Metric/Imperial		American
180g/6oz	brown basmati rice	¾ cup
2 tbs	tomato purée/tomato paste	2 tbs
Scant 300ml/½ pint	vegetable stock	1⅓ cups
120g/4oz	sweetcorn, canned and drained	⅔ cup
60g/2oz	frozen garden peas	⅓ cup
120g/4oz	carrot, finely diced	1 large

1. Wash the rice under cold running water, put it into a bowl, cover with cold water and leave it to soak for 20–30 minutes.
2. Mix the tomato purée (tomato paste) with the stock, pour into a saucepan and add the sweetcorn and frozen peas.
3. Drain the rice, then stir the rice and diced carrot into the saucepan.
4. Bring the mixture to the boil, reduce the heat and stir well. Cover the saucepan and leave it over a low heat for 20 minutes.

5. Remove the lid from the saucepan and stir. The grains of rice should be fluffy and separate. If necessary, cook the mixture for a further 2 minutes until all the stock has been absorbed.

Note to Cooks

Not suitable for freezing.

SAVOURY RICE PUDDING

This unusual dish can be eaten hot or cold. For the less adventurous, the recipe can be served after step 3, but do not stir the cheese in with the fruit and nuts, just crumble it over the top.

Serves 4

Metric/Imperial		American
1½ tsp	olive oil	1½ tsp
90g/3oz	onion, finely chopped	½ cup
180g/6oz	long-grain brown rice, e.g., basmati	¾ cup
105g/3½oz	blue Stilton, crumbled into small pieces	⅞ cup
60g/2oz	dry-roasted peanuts	3½ tbs
30g/1oz	raisins	⅛ cup
90g/3oz	apple, cored and chopped	½ cup

1. Heat the oil in a saucepan, add the onion and stir-fry for about 5 minutes.
2. Stir the rice into the saucepan and then cook according to the directions on the pack in the recommended amount of liquid until the grains are fluffy and separate.
3. Stir the cheese, nuts and fruit into the hot rice and continue to stir until the cheese has melted.
4. Lightly grease a 600ml (1 pint/½ quart) ring mould (tube pan), spoon the rice mixture into the mould and press it down firmly so the surface is level.

5. Bake the pudding at 325°F/160°C/gas mark 3 for 5–6 minutes.
6. Remove the Savoury Rice Pudding from the oven, invert the mould onto a serving plate, tap sharply, then lift off the mould.

Note to Cooks

Not suitable for freezing.

MELBA TOAST

Melba Toast is served with a number of dishes, such as pâté and dips. It is usually made from refined white bread, but wholemeal (wholewheat) toast adds flavour as well as fibre.

Serves 4

Metric/Imperial		American
12	very thin slices of wholemeal/wholewheat bread	12

1. Remove the crusts from the bread. The total weight of the slices should be about 120g (4oz).
2. Cut each slice in half to make 2 triangles.
3. Put the triangles of bread on the rack of a grill (broiler) pan and cook under low to moderate heat until they are golden brown. Turn and cook the other side. (Alternatively, cook the bread on a baking tray (baking sheet) in a moderate oven until it is dry and golden brown.) The Melba Toast should curl slightly and be a fairly even colour when it is cooked.

Handy hint: If, like many people, you find it difficult to cut thin enough slices, try the following method.

Cut 6 thicker slices, remove crusts and toast on both sides. Then cut each slice in half to expose the untoasted centres. You now have 12 slices of toast, which can be cut into triangles and toasted as normal.

Note to Cooks
Not suitable for freezing.

YORKSHIRE PUDDING

This recipe is made by a completely different method from the traditional Yorkshire Pudding, yet the result is really light.

Serves 4

Metric/Imperial		American
120g/4oz	plain/all-purpose brown flour	1 cup
2	eggs	2
1 tbs	sunflower oil	1 tbs
270ml/9 fl oz	milk	generous cup

1. Preheat the oven to 425°F/220°C/gas mark 7.
2. Sieve (sift) the flour into a bowl and make a well in the centre.
3. Separate the eggs and drop the yolks into the well and the whites into a clean bowl.
4. Spoon the oil into an ovenproof dish about 28 × 22.5 × 5cm (11 × 9 × 2 in), tipping the dish so that the oil coats the base, then put the dish in the hot oven while completing the recipe.
5. Pour about half the milk into the well in the bowl of flour, then gradually beat the egg yolks and milk into the flour. When the mixture is a smooth, creamy consistency, beat in the remaining milk.
6. Whisk the egg whites until they form soft peaks. Gently fold the egg whites into the batter.

7. Spoon the batter into the hot dish and bake for 35–40 minutes until it has risen well and is brown and crisp. Serve immediately.

Note to Cooks

Not suitable for freezing.

BANANA TEABREAD

This teabread freezes well and may be frozen as a whole loaf or in slices.

Serves 12

Metric/Imperial		American
240g/8oz	wholemeal/wholewheat flour	2 cups
2½ tsp	baking powder	2½ tsp
90g/3oz	margarine	⅓ cup
90g/3oz	demerara/raw brown or caster/superfine sugar	⅓ cup
60g/2oz	walnuts/English walnuts, roughly chopped	½ cup
2	eggs, beaten	2

1. Lightly grease and line a 19 × 11.5cm (7½ × 4½ in) loaf tin (pan).
2. Sieve (sift) the flour and baking powder into a bowl. Tip the bran remaining in the sieve (sifter) into the bowl.
3. In a separate bowl, cream (beat) the margarine and sugar together.
4. Peel and mash the bananas then stir into the creamed mixture.
5. Add the walnuts (English walnuts) and eggs, stir well, then gradually mix in the flour.
6. Spoon the mixture into the prepared tin (pan), level the surface and bake at 350°F/180°C/gas mark 4 for

1 hour and 10 minutes until it has risen and is firm to the touch.

7. Leave the teabread to cool in the tin (pan) for 20 minutes, then turn it out (unmold it), remove the paper and transfer it to a cooling rack until it is cold. Store for 24 hours before slicing.

CARROT BUNS

Carrots add moisture and sweetness to recipes and this recipe makes full use of both these qualities.

Serves 10

Metric/Imperial		*American*
180g/6oz	wholemeal/wholewheat flour	1½ cups
30g/1oz	fine oatmeal	3 tbs
2 tsp	bicarbonate of soda/ baking soda	2 tsp
60g/2oz	margarine	¼ cup
45g/1½oz	pecan kernels	⅜ cup
45g/1½oz	soft brown sugar	3 tbs
60g/2oz	dried mixed fruit	⅓ cup
90g/3oz	carrot, coarsely grated	1 medium
1	egg, lightly beaten	1
3–4 tbs	milk	3–4 tbs

1. Lightly grease 10 patty tins (muffin pans) or 2 baking trays (baking sheets).
2. Sieve (sift) the flour, oatmeal and bicarbonate of soda (baking soda) into a bowl. Tip the bran remaining in the sieve (sifter) into the bowl.
3. Rub (cut) the margarine into the flour until the mixture resembles fine breadcrumbs.
4. Reserve 10 pecans. Finely chop the remainder then stir into the flour mixture together with the sugar, dried fruit and carrot.

5. Pour the egg and 3 tbs of the milk into the flour mixture and mix with a fork to form a mixture that will drop from the fork when gently tapped on the edge of the bowl. Add a little more milk if necessary.

6. Spoon the mixture into the prepared tins (pans) or put 10 spoonfuls of the mixture onto the baking trays (baking sheets) and roughen the tops with a fork. Gently press a reserved pecan half into each Bun.

7. Bake the Buns at 400°F/200°C/gas mark 6 for 20–25 minutes. Leave in the tins (pans) for a few minutes to cool a little, then transfer them to a cooling rack.

DATE CAKE

This cake is simple to make and keeps well.

Serves 10

Metric/Imperial		*American*
300g/10oz	self-raising wholemeal/ self-rising wholewheat flour	2½ cups
300g/10oz	stoned (pitted) dried dates	2 cups
150ml/5 fl oz	sunflower or corn oil	⅔ cup
	finely grated zest and juice of an orange	
1	egg, lightly beaten	1

1. Grease and line a 17.5 × 10cm (7 × 4 in) loaf tin (pan) with non-stick baking paper (baking parchment) or greaseproof paper (waxed paper).
2. Sieve (sift) the flour into a bowl. Tip the bran remaining in the sieve (sifter) into the bowl.
3. Finely chop 180g (6oz) dates and stir into the flour. Roughly chop the remaining dates, checking that there aren't any stones (pits) in them, then put them into a liquidizer (blender).
4. Pour the oil into the liquidizer (blender) and process until a purée has been formed.
5. Stir the orange zest into the flour and date mixture.
6. Pour the orange juice into a measuring jug and add sufficient water to make up to 180ml (6 fl oz/¾ cup).

7. Pour the juice and water into the liquidizer (blender) and process once again until well combined.
8. Stir the egg and the blended mixture into the flour and dates and mix well with a wooden spoon.
9. Transfer the mixture to the prepared tin (pan) level the surface and bake at 350°F/180°C/gas mark 4 for 1 hour 10 minutes. Leave to cool for 15 minutes then turn out (unmold), removing the lining paper, and transfer to a cooling rack.

STICKY FRUIT BUNS

When preparing any yeast mixture, warm all the ingredients to speed up the rising process. If you prefer to use dried yeast in place of fresh, follow the manufacturer's directions as to quantities. Unless otherwise stated, dissolve the yeast and ½ teaspoon of sugar in the warm liquid and leave for 10–15 minutes until it becomes frothy, then continue from step 2.

Serves 10

Metric/Imperial		American
15g/½ oz	fresh yeast	1¼ tbs
Approx. 210ml/7 fl oz	warm milk (hand hot, not boiling)	Approx. ¾ cup
480g/1 lb	wholemeal/wholewheat flour	4 cups
1½ tsp	salt	1½ tsp
1 tbs	soft brown sugar	1 tbs
60g/2oz	margarine	¼ cup
120g/4oz	dried mixed fruit	⅔ cup
1	egg, lightly beaten	1

For the glaze

2 tbs	soft brown sugar	2 tbs
4 tbs	water	4 tbs

1. Crumble the yeast into a jug and gradually blend in 210ml (7 fl oz/¾ cup) of the warm milk.
2. Sieve (sift) the flour and salt into a bowl. Tip the

bran remaining in the sieve (sifter) into the bowl.

3. Stir in the sugar and rub (cut) in the margarine until it resembles breadcrumbs.

4. Stir in the dried fruit, then make a well in the centre of the mixture.

5. Pour the egg into the well and then the yeast liquid. Mix everything together well until you have an elastic dough (add a little more warm milk if it is too dry).

6. Lightly flour a work surface and knead the dough by drawing up about one-third of it with your knuckles and pressing it down onto the remaining two-thirds, then pressing it with the palms of your hands in a rhythmic action. Knead for about 10 minutes until the dough is smooth and elastic.

7. Put the dough in a clean bowl, cover with a lightly greased piece of polythene or clingfilm (saran wrap) and leave it in a warm place for about 40 minutes until it has doubled in size.

8. Knead the dough once again, divide it into 10 pieces and shape into buns.

9. Put the buns on 2 lightly greased baking trays (baking sheets) leaving a little space between them, cover with the lightly greased polythene or clingfilm (saran wrap) and leave in a warm place for about 30 minutes until they have almost doubled in size.

10. Bake the buns at 450°F/230°C/gas mark 8 for 15–20 minutes until they are golden brown and, when lightly tapped on the base, they sound slightly hollow. Transfer them to a rack to cool.

11. Make the glaze by gently heating the sugar and water in a small saucepan. When the sugar has dissolved, increase the heat and boil rapidly for 1–2 minutes. Brush the buns with the hot glaze and leave until cold.

EGGLESS FRUIT CAKE

The proportions of the dried fruits can be varied as long as the total weight remains the same.

Makes 12 slices

Metric/Imperial		American
540ml/18 fl oz	pineapple juice	2¼ cups
120g/4oz	dried stoned (pitted) dates, chopped	⅔ cup
90g/3oz	dried figs, chopped	⅔ cup
90g/3oz	chopped mixed peel	½ cup
120g/4oz	sultanas/golden seedless raisins or raisins	⅔ cup
180g/6oz	soft brown sugar	1 cup
180g/6oz	margarine	¾ cup
450g/1 lb	wholemeal/wholewheat flour	4 cups
2 tbs	baking powder	2 tbs
1 tsp	bicarbonate of soda/ baking soda	1 tsp

1. Grease and line a 20cm (8 in) round very deep cake tin (pan).
2. Pour the pineapple juice into a saucepan, add all the fruits, sugar and margarine and bring to the boil. Reduce the heat and simmer for 10 minutes, then remove from the heat and leave to cool for 30 minutes.
3. Sieve (sift) the flour, baking powder and bicarbonate of soda (baking soda) into a bowl. Tip the bran remaining in the sieve (sifter) into the bowl.

Irritable Bowel Syndrome

4. Pour the pineapple juice and fruit mixture into the bowl and mix well.
5. Spoon the mixture into the prepared tin (pan) and level the top.
6. Bake at 350°F/180°C/gas mark 4 for 11/2 hours. Leave to cool in the tin (pan) for 30–40 minutes then turn out (unmold) and transfer to a cooling rack.

YEAST CAKE

This recipe is for the more experienced cook who is used to handling yeast mixtures. It is important to use warm ingredients, so put the flour and dried fruit into a warm cupboard well before making the recipe. If you prefer, use dried yeast in place of fresh, following the manufacturer's directions regarding quantities. Unless otherwise stated, dissolve the yeast and ½ teaspoon sugar in the warm liquid and leave in a warm place for 10–15 minutes until it becomes frothy then continue from step 2.

Serves 12

Metric/Imperial		American
Just under 20g/¾oz	fresh yeast	scant 2 tbs
360ml/12 fl oz	warm milk	1½ cups
600g/1 lb 4oz	wholemeal/wholewheat flour	5 cups
1½ tsp	salt	1½ tsp
15g/½ oz	soft brown sugar	1 tbs
90g/3oz	margarine	⅓ cup
300g/10oz	dried mixed fruit	1⅔ cup
2 tsp	clear honey	2 tsp

1. Crumble the yeast into a jug and gradually blend in 300ml (½ pint/1¼ cups) of the warm milk.
2. Sieve (sift) the flour and salt into a bowl. Tip the bran remaining in the sieve (sifter) into the bowl.

3. Stir in the sugar and rub (cut) in the margarine until the mixture resembles breadcrumbs.

4. Make a well in the centre of the mixture, pour in the yeast liquid and mix to form a soft dough until the dough leaves the sides of the bowl. Add extra warm milk if the mixture is still too dry.

5. Transfer the dough to a lightly floured work surface and knead by drawing about one-third of the dough up with your knuckles and folding it back onto the remaining two-thirds, then pressing down firmly with the palms of your hands in a rhythmic movement for about 10 minutes, until it becomes stiff and smooth.

6. Put the dough into a clean bowl, cover with a lightly greased piece of polythene or clingfilm (saran wrap) and leave in a warm place for about 1 hour until it has doubled in size.

7. Knead the dough once again, then gradually knead in the warm dried fruit —persevering even when the fruit keeps springing out!

8. Lightly grease a 20cm (8 in) round cake tin (pan) and put the dough into the tin (pan), pressing it firmly into place. Cover with lightly greased polythene or cling-film (saran wrap) and leave it in a warm place until well risen.

9. Bake the Yeast Cake at 425°F/220°C/gas mark 7 for 40 minutes until cooked. Turn the cake out of the tin (pan) and gently tap the base: if it sounds hollow, it is cooked; if not, return to the oven for a few more minutes.

10. Transfer the cooked cake to a cooling rack.
11. Meanwhile, pour the honey into a cup or small bowl and stand in a saucepan of simmering water until it becomes runny, then brush it over the warm cake and leave it to finish cooling.

SIMPLE MALT LOAF

This loaf has an interesting texture and remains deliciously moist for several days.

Makes 12 slices

Metric/Imperial		American
225g/8oz	wholemeal/wholewheat flour	2 cups
1¼ tsp	bicarbonate of soda/ baking soda	1¼ tsp
30g/1oz	bran	¼ cup
240ml/8 fl oz	milk	1 cup
60g/2oz	golden syrup/corn syrup	¼ cup
60g/2oz	malt	¼ cup
120g/4oz	sultanas/golden seedless raisins	⅔ cup

1. Lightly grease and line a 19 × 11.5cm (7½ × 4½ in) loaf tin (pan).
2. Sieve (sift) the flour and bicarbonate of soda (baking soda) into a bowl. Tip the bran remaining in the sieve (sifter) into the bowl, then stir in the additional bran.
3. Reserve 150ml (5 fl oz/⅔ cup) of the milk, pour the remainder into a small saucepan and add the syrup and malt. Stir gently over a very low heat until the syrup, malt and milk are well mixed but only just warm.
4. Pour the reserved milk and the syrup mixture into the flour, mix well, add the sultanas (golden seedless raisins) and stir round once again.

5. Spoon the mixture into the lined tin (pan) and level the top.
6. Bake at 325°F/160°C/gas mark 3 for about 1 hour 10 minutes, or until firm and a warm skewer, when inserted into the middle of the loaf, comes out clean.
7. Remove the loaf from the oven and leave to cool in the tin (pan) for 15 minutes then turn out (unmold), remove the paper and leave on a cooling rack. Store for 24 hours before cutting.

WHOLESOME CARROT CAKE

The combination of wholemeal (wholewheat) flour, dried fruits and carrots provides a valuable source of dietary fibre, far more than would a cake made from refined white flour.

Serves 10

Metric/Imperial		American
180ml/6 fl oz	clear honey	¾ cup
120ml/4 fl oz	corn or safflower oil	½ cup
225g/8oz	wholemeal/wholewheat flour	2 cups
1 tbs	baking powder	1 tbs
90g/3oz	dried stoned/pitted dates, chopped	½ cups
90g/3oz	sultanas/golden seedless raisins	½ cup
2	eggs, lightly beaten	2
2 tbs	frozen concentrated orange juice, thawed	2 tbs
225g/8oz	carrots, finely grated	2 large

1. Lightly grease a 20cm (8 in) round cake tin (pan) and line it with non-stick baking paper (baking parchment).
2. Pour the honey into a small saucepan and heat gently until it is very runny – but just to this point, do not overheat. Remove the pan from the heat and stir in the oil.

Cereal recipes

3. Sieve (sift) the flour and baking powder into a bowl. Tip the bran remaining in the sieve (sifter) into the bowl.
4. Stir the dates and sultanas (golden seedless raisins) into the flour.
5. Make a well in the centre of the dry ingredients, pour half the cooled honey and oil, the eggs and orange juice into it and beat all the ingredients together well.
6. Gradually add the remaining honey and oil and stir in the carrots.
7. Pour the cake mixture into the prepared tin (pan) and bake at 350°F/180°C/gas mark 4 for about 1½ hours until level, golden brown and firm to the touch.
8. Leave the carrot cake in the tin (pan) for 30 minutes then turn it out (unmold) onto a wire rack and leave it to cool.

APRICOT SEMOLINA

This pudding is very simple to make.

Serves 2

Metric/Imperial		American
60g/2oz	wholemeal/wholewheat semolina	½ cup
600ml/1 pint	milk	2½ cups
120g/4oz	no-soak dried apricots, chopped	¾ cup
120g/4oz	fromage frais	½ cup
1–2 tsp	honey	1–2 tsp

1. Spoon the semolina into a saucepan and gradually blend in the milk, then add the apricots.
2. Bring the semolina mixture to the boil, stirring all the time, and boil for 3–4 minutes, stirring occasionally, until it is thick.
3. Leave the semolina to cool for a few minutes, then spoon it and the fromage frais into a liquidizer (blender) and process to a smooth purée.
4. Sweeten the purée with a little honey – don't over-sweeten it or the flavour will be spoilt.
5. Spoon the Apricot Semolina into 4 glasses and leave until cold.

BREAD PUDDING

This pudding may be served hot, with custard or yogurt, or if you prefer, serve cold.

Serves 4

Metric/Imperial		*American*
180g/6oz	wholemeal/wholewheat bread	5 slices
300ml/½ pint	milk	1⅓ cups
45g/1½oz	margarine	3 tbs
3 tbs	frozen concentrated orange juice, thawed	3 tbs
30g/1oz	soft brown sugar	2 tbs
1	egg, lightly beaten	1
180g/6oz	dried mixed fruit	1 cup

1. Lightly grease a 900ml (1½ pint/¾ quart) pie dish.
2. Break the bread into small pieces then put into a bowl.
3. Heat the milk until steaming, pour it over the bread and leave it to soak for 30 minutes.
4. Melt the margarine in a small saucepan.
5. Beat the soaked bread with a wooden spoon until smooth, mix in all the remaining ingredients.
6. Spoon the mixture into the pie dish and bake at 350°F/180°C/gas mark 4 for 1¼ to 1½ hours.

FRUIT AND BREAD BAKE

Use really good wholemeal (wholewheat) bread, such as
the Short Time Wholemeal Bread (see page 98 for recipe).

Serves 4

Metric/Imperial		American
2 tsp	margarine	2 tsp
5 thin slices	wholemeal/wholewheat bread	5 thin slices
1 tbs	pear 'n'apple spread	1 tbs
50g/2oz	dried apple, finely chopped	½ cup
450ml/¾ pint	milk	2 cups
2	eggs, lightly beaten	2

1. Lightly grease a 900ml (1½ pint/¾ quart) pie dish with
   a little of the margarine.
2. Spread 2 slices of bread with the remaining margarine.
   Spread the other slices with the pear 'n' apple spread.
3. Cut the bread into strips.
4. Arrange half the strips of bread with the fruit spread-
   side uppermost over the base of the pie dish. Sprinkle
   half the apple into the dish, cover with the remaining
   bread, then sprinkle the rest of the apple over the top.
5. Heat the milk until steaming, then whisk (beat) in the
   eggs. Strain the milk and egg mixture over the bread
   and leave it to soak in for 20 minutes.
6. Cook at 350°F/180°C/gas mark 4 for 30–40 minutes.

Notes to Cooks
Not suitable for freezing.

FRUITY BREAD PUDDING

This is a variation on the traditional bread-and-butter pudding, but it doesn't have its crunchy top and contains no added fat.

Serves 4

Metric/Imperial		American
90g/3oz	fresh wholemeal/ wholewheat breadcrumbs	1½ cups
90g/3oz	dried mixed fruit	½ cup
300ml/½ pint	milk	1⅓ cup
15g/½ oz	sugar	1 tbs
½	lemon, finely grated zest of	½
1	egg, lightly beaten	1

1. Mix the breadcrumbs with the dried fruit then spread them evenly into a 600ml (1 pint/½ quart) ovenproof dish.
2. Pour the milk into a small saucepan. Add the sugar and lemon zest and heat until the milk is steaming and the sugar has dissolved.
3. Pour the milk mixture over the egg, mix well, then pour this mixture over the breadcrumb and fruit mixture and leave to stand for 20 minutes.
4. Bake at 350°F/180°C/gas mark 4 for 35–40 minutes until set. Serve hot or cold.

Note to Cooks

Not suitable for freezing.

PANCAKES (CRÊPES)

Pancakes (crêpes) made with purely wholemeal (wholewheat) flour tend to be stodgy, but this mixture of white and wholemeal (wholewheat) flour gives a good result. If possible use a non-stick frying pan (skillet) so that you can reduce the amount of oil required for cooking.

Serves 4

Metric/Imperial		American
60g/2oz	plain/all-purpose white flour	½ cup
60g/2oz	wholemeal/wholewheat flour	½ cup
1 large	egg	1 extra large
300ml/½ pint	milk	1⅓ cups
	salt	
	oil	

1. Sieve (sift) the flours into a bowl. Tip the bran left in the sieve (sifter) into the flour, and make a well in the centre.
2. Break the egg into the well, add about half the milk and, using a wooden spoon or whisk (beater), beat the egg and milk together in the well, drawing the flour gradually into the liquid. When smooth, stir in the remaining milk.
3. To make thin pancakes (crêpes), all frying pans (skillets), unless they are non-stick, must be proved as this

enables the batter to cook in very little oil and so helps to prevent it sticking. To prove the pan, tip about 1 tbs of salt into the frying pan (skillet) and put it over a low heat until the salt is hot. Tip the salt out and remove the pan from the heat. Allow to cool, then wipe round the inside of the pan with a wad of kitchen paper (paper towels). Add a little oil to the frying pan (skillet), heat it gently, then remove from the heat and wipe once again with a pad of kitchen paper (paper towels).

4. Add a little oil to the pan and heat gently, tipping the frying pan (skillet) slightly so the oil just covers its base. Tip the frying pan (skillet) with one hand while pouring in just enough batter to coat its base. Cook over a moderate heat until the underside is golden, then toss or turn the pancake (crêpe) and cook the other side.

5. Slide the cooked pancake (crêpe) onto a plate, cover and keep warm in a low oven while cooking the remaining batter. This mixture will make about 14 × 15cm (6 in) pancakes (crêpes).

6. Serve hot with lemon, drizzled with a little honey, or with a sweet or savoury filling.

7

Fruit and vegetable recipes

Savoury
Avocado with Blue Cheese
Baked Potato
   with Baked Beans
   with Coleslaw
Bean Salad
Carrot Salad
Carrot and Parsnip Salad
Chunky Tomato Sauce
Coleslaw
Cucumber Salad
Date and Pineapple Salad
Fishy Potato Salad
Fruitslaw
Fruity Beetroot (Beets)
Leek and Watercress Soup
Minestrone
Parsnip Soup with Apple
Potato Salad
Ratatouille
Savoury Banana Salad
Simple Vegetable Soup
Springtime Salad
Stir-fried Vegetables

Stuffed Mushrooms
Stuffed Tomatoes
Summer Salad
Sweetcorn and Peas
Vegetable Barley
   Casserole
Whole Tomato Salad

Sweet
Bramble Brown Betty
Creamy-topped Fruit
Dried Fruit Compote
Fresh Fruit Jelly
Fruit Bars
Fruitels
Fruity Cheese Ring
Oatmeal Ambrosia
Peaches with Raspberries
Stuffed Apples
Summer Sundae
Sweet Date Pancakes
   (Crêpes)
Winter Fruit Salad

AVOCADO WITH BLUE CHEESE

If you are making this recipe for a dinner party, use a selection of different varieties of lettuce to make a colourful, sophisticated base for the avocado.

Serves 4

Metric/Imperial		American
45g/1½oz	Danish blue cheese, crumbled	⅜ cup
4 tbs	buttermilk	4 tbs
1 tsp	lemon juice	1 tsp
1 large	tomato	1 large
45g/1½oz	small black olives, stoned/pitted	15
1 large	avocado	1
4 large	lettuce leaves	4
	Melba Toast (see page 124)	

1. Mash the blue cheese until smooth, then gradually mix in the buttermilk and ½ tsp of the lemon juice.
2. Cover the tomato with boiling water, leave for 30–40 seconds, then drain and slip off the skin. Halve the tomato, scoop out the seeds and cut the flesh into 1.25cm (½ in) pieces.
3. Put the olives in a bowl.
4. Halve the avocado, remove the stone (pit) and peel. Cut the avocado into 1.2 to 2cm (½ to ¾ in) cubes. Add to the olives.

5. Mix the avocado together with the tomato and olives, sprinkle the remaining lemon juice over them and stir round gently to coat all the ingredients well.
6. Arrange the lettuce leaves on 4 small serving plates, spoon the avocado mixture onto each leaf and spoon the blue cheese dressing over the top. Serve with the Melba Toast.

Note to Cooks

Not suitable for freezing.

BAKED POTATO

If you own a microwave, the potatoes may be cooked very quickly, but the skin will not have the same crispness as those baked in a conventional oven.

Serves 1

Metric/Imperial		American
180g/6oz	potato	1 medium
1 tbs	natural/plain yogurt (optional)	1 tbs
1 tsp	chives, chopped (optional)	1 tsp

1. Scrub the potato well, then prick it all over with a fork or cut a cross on its top side.
2. If you are baking it in a conventional oven, insert a skewer through the potato to speed up the cooking. Bake between 180 and 200°C /350–400°F/gas mark 4–6 for 50–60 minutes until cooked.
3. Serve the potato on its own or cut a cross into the top, open it up and spoon the yogurt, mixed with the chives, into the centre.

Note to Cooks

Not suitable for freezing.

VARIATIONS

Serves 1

Metric/Imperial   *American*

Baked potato with baked beans

180g/6oz	potato	1 medium
120g/4oz	baked beans	½ cup

1. and 2. As 1. and 2. of Baked Potatoes opposite.
3. Halve the cooked potato then spoon baked beans on top.

Note to Cooks

Not suitable for freezing.

Baked Potato with Coleslaw

Serves 1

180g/6oz	potato	1 medium
¼ quantity	Coleslaw (see page 161)	¼ quantity

1. and 2. As 1. and 2. of Baked Potato opposite.
3. Cut a cross into the top of the potato, open it up and spoon the Coleslaw into the centre.

Note to Cooks

Not suitable for freezing.

BEAN SALAD

The combination of textures and flavours makes this salad an ideal accompaniment to fish, meat, cheese or eggs. It could also be served as the main protein component of a meal, making a tasty vegetarian option.

Serves 4

Metric/Imperial		*American*
90g/3oz	dwarf French/fine green beans	¾ cup
270g/9oz	kidney beans, canned and drained or dried and freshly cooked	1½ cups
90g/3oz	bean sprouts	1½ cups
120g/4oz	tomatoes	2 small
2 tsp	tomato purée/tomato paste	2 tsp
1 tbs	wine vinegar	1 tbs
1½ tbs	olive oil	1½ tbs
1 tsp	chives, chopped	1 tsp

1. Cut the French beans (fine green beans) into 4cm (1½ in) lengths, cook in boiling water for 7–8 minutes, until just tender, then drain well.
2. Mix the French beans (fine green beans) with the kidney beans and bean sprouts.
3. Put the tomatoes into a bowl, cover with boiling water, leave for 30–40 seconds, then drain and slip off their skins. Cut each tomato in half, scoop out and discard the seeds, then roughly chop the tomato flesh.

4. Whisk the tomato purée (tomato paste) with the vinegar, oil and chives.
5. Pour the dressing over the beans and mix well.

Note to Cooks

Not suitable for freezing.

CARROT SALAD

The tang of the oranges complements the sweetness of the carrots and dried fruit to make a refreshing salad.

Serves 4

Metric/Imperial		American
2	oranges	2
45g/1½oz	sultanas/golden seedless raisins or raisins	2 tbs
180g/6oz	carrots, coarsely grated	2 medium

1. Squeeze out the juice of half of one of the oranges.
2. Put the dried fruit into a bowl, add the orange juice and leave for several hours or overnight.
3. Remove the peel and white pith from the remaining half and second orange. Roughly chop them, saving any juice that runs from the fruit.
4. Mix the chopped oranges with the carrots, soaked fruit and any remaining orange juice.

Note to Cooks

Not suitable for freezing.

CARROT AND PARSNIP SALAD

A food processor with a grater attachment is an ideal and labour-saving way to prepare the vegetables.

Serves 4

Metric/Imperial		American
180g/6oz	carrots, finely grated	2 medium
180g/6oz	parsnips, finely grated	2 medium
30g/1oz	sultanas/golden seedless raisins	1 tbs
1 tbs	grapeseed or olive oil	1 tbs
1 small	orange, juice of	1 small
3–4 tsp	finely chopped coriander/cilantro	3–4 tsp

1. Put the carrot and parsnip into a bowl and stir in the sultanas (golden seedless raisins).
2. Put the oil, orange juice and coriander (cilantro) into a small bowl and whisk (beat) until evenly combined.
3. Pour the dressing over the salad and stir well. Chill until ready to serve. Stir again before serving to ensure the dressing evenly coats the salad.

Note to Cooks

Not suitable for freezing.

CHUNKY TOMATO SAUCE

Make this sauce in summer when tomatoes are cheap, plentiful and full of flavour. Freeze it in quantities to use throughout the winter.

Makes about 750ml
(1¼ pints/3½ cups) to serve 8

Metric/Imperial		American
1kg/2 lb	tomatoes	2 lb
1 tbs	olive oil	1 tbs
120g/4oz	onion, finely chopped	1
60g/2oz	carrot, grated	1 small
1 tbs	finely chopped basil	1 tbs
1 tbs	tomato purée/tomato paste	1 tbs

1. Cover the tomatoes with boiling water, leave them for 30–40 seconds, then drain and slip off the skins. (Don't try to do this with all the tomatoes in one bowl, otherwise the water will cool too quickly and the skins won't slip off.)
2. Roughly chop the tomatoes, put them and all the other ingredients into a saucepan and stir well. Cover the saucepan and leave over a moderate heat for 30 minutes, stirring occasionally.
3. Remove the saucepan lid, stir the sauce and leave to simmer uncovered for 30 minutes until thick. Serve as a hot sauce or as a topping for cooked recipes such as cannelloni.

COLESLAW

This salad can be prepared in a few minutes if you use a food processor but, if you don't have one, it will take quite a while to prepare. This coleslaw retains its texture far better than the prepared salad sold in many supermarkets.

Serves 4

Metric/Imperial		American
180g/6oz	white cabbage	⅓ small
120g/4oz	carrot	1 large
15g/½ oz	onion	¼ small
60g/2oz	sticks/stalks celery	2 medium
3 tbs	mayonnaise	3 tbs
5 tbs	low-fat natural/plain yogurt	5 tbs

1. Finely shred or coarsely grate the white cabbage.
2. Coarsely grate the carrot and onion.
3. Finely chop the celery.
4. Mix the white cabbage together with the carrot, celery and onion.
5. Add the mayonnaise and yogurt and stir until all the ingredients are well combined. (*Note* If the Coleslaw is prepared a few hours before it is to be eaten, stir it well just before you serve it so that the dressing evenly coats the vegetables.)

Note to Cooks

Not suitable for freezing.

CUCUMBER SALAD

Serve this refreshing salad with a variety of other salads – this will increase the overall fibre content of the meal.

Serves 4

Metric/Imperial		*American*
120g/4oz	cucumber	4 in piece
½ small or	canteloupe or honeydew	½ small or
¼ large	melon	¼ large
6 large	radishes	6 large

1. Cut the cucumber into 1.2cm (½ in) dice and put them into a bowl.
2. Scoop out and discard the seeds from the melon, remove the skin and then cut the flesh into 1.2cm (½ in) dice.
3. Cut each radish into quarters.
4. Add the melon and radishes to the cucumber and mix well. Serve as soon as possible.

Note to Cooks

Not suitable for freezing.

DATE AND PINEAPPLE SALAD

The refreshing mixture of fromage frais and orange juice gives an additional tang to the mixture of dates and pineapple.

Serves 4

Metric/Imperial		American
8	fresh dates	8
300g/10oz	fresh pineapple, cubed	2 cups
90g/3oz	fromage frais	½ cup
1 tbs	frozen concentrated orange juice, thawed	1 tbs

1. Cut the dates in half and remove the stones (pits), then cut each date in half again.
2. Stir the fromage frais into the orange juice, then pour over the pineapple and dates and mix well.

Note to Cooks

Not suitable for freezing.

FISHY POTATO SALAD

The firm, waxy texture of new potatoes is ideal for this tasty alternative to a plain potato salad.

Serves 6

Metric/Imperial		American
720g/1½ lb	new potatoes	1½ lb
small		small
	sprig of mint	
50g/1¾oz	canned anchovy fillets in oil	10
1 tbs	olive or sunflower oil	1 tbs
4 tsp	wine vinegar	4 tsp
4 tsp	chopped mint	4 tsp
2–4 tsp	chopped chives	2–4 tsp

1. Scrub the potatoes well, then put into a saucepan of boiling water with the mint. Cover the saucepan and cook for 12–15 minutes until they are cooked but firm.
2. Drain the oil from the anchovy fillets into a small bowl and put the fillets to one side.
3. Add the olive or sunflower oil to the bowl and mix in the vinegar, mint and chives.
4. Drain the hot potatoes and put them into a bowl, discard the sprig of mint.
5. Whisk the oil mixture then pour over the hot potatoes.
6. Cut the anchovy fillets in half along their length then in half across their width. Stir the anchovy fillets into the potato salad and leave until completely cold.

Note to Cooks
Not suitable for freezing.

FRUITSLAW

This recipe is a mixture of a coleslaw, savoury fruit and Waldorf salad all rolled into one! Make sure you drain the canned fruits well or the liquid will sink to the bottom of the serving dish. Use fruit that is tinned (canned) in unsweetened natural juice.

Serves 6

Metric/Imperial		*American*
300g/10oz	white cabbage	⅔ small
180g/6oz	carrots	2 medium
2	sticks/stalks celery	2
30g/1oz	walnuts/English walnuts, roughly chopped	3 tbs
30g/1oz	no-soak dried apricots, chopped	2 tbs
30g/1oz	raisins	3 tbs
90g/3oz	canned mandarins, well drained	½ cup
90g/3oz	canned pineapple, well drained and chopped	½ cup
5 tbs	mayonnaise	5 tbs
4 tbs	natural/plain yogurt	4 tbs

1. Finely shred the white cabbage, carrots and celery. (This is done quickly in a food processor with a shredding attachment, but if you prefer, use a very sharp knife to cut the cabbage and celery as thinly as possible, then grate the carrots.)

2. Mix the cabbage, carrots and celery together in a bowl, then add the walnuts (English walnuts), apricots, raisins, mandarins and pineapple.
3. Blend the mayonnaise with the yogurt then add to the bowl and stir it through the salad. (*Note* If the Fruitslaw is to be kept for a few hours or overnight, cover the bowl with clingfilm (saran wrap) and stir it well just before serving.)

Note to Cooks

Not suitable for freezing.

FRUITY BEETROOT (BEETS)

The sharp flavours of the grapefruit and orange combine well with the beetroot (beets) to make a tasty salad.

Serves 4

Metric/Imperial		American
360g/12oz	beetroot/beets, freshly cooked	10 small
½	grapefruit	½
1	orange	1
1 tbs	chopped parsley	1 tbs

1. Remove the skins from the beetroot (beets), cut flesh into thick slices, then cut the slices into short, thick lengths.
2. Peel the grapefruit and orange, divide them into segments, then cut each segment into 2 or 3 pieces.
3. Mix the beetroot (beets) with the fruit and parsley.

Note to Cooks

Not suitable for freezing.

LEEK AND WATERCRESS SOUP

This soup, served with crusty wholemeal (wholewheat) bread, makes a delicious snack lunch for 4 people, but if you wish to serve it as part of a three-course meal, simply serve 6 slightly smaller portions.

Serves 4

Metric/Imperial		*American*
240g/8oz	leeks	2 cups
60g/2oz	watercress	2 cups
1 tbs	margarine	1 tbs
300g/10oz	potatoes, chopped	1⅔ cups
450ml/¾ pint	stock	2 cups
180ml/6 fl oz	milk	⅔ cup

1. Slice the leeks and roughly chop the watercress.
2. Heat the margarine in a saucepan, add the leeks and stir-fry for 2–3 minutes. Stir the watercress into the saucepan, cover and place over a low heat for 8 minutes.
3. Add the potatoes, stir, then add the stock, cover and leave to simmer for 25–30 minutes.
4. Pour the soup into a liquidizer (blender) or food processor and process to a purée.
5. Pour the soup back into the saucepan and stir in the milk. Reheat the soup and, if necessary, add a little more milk. Ladle into warm bowls.

MINESTRONE

This recipe is very adaptable, other vegetables can be included if desired. Use freshly grated Parmesan cheese – it has a much better flavour than the pre-grated packaged Parmesan.

Serves 6

Metric/Imperial		American
60g/2oz	dried haricot/navy beans	¼ cup
3 rashers	streaky bacon	3 slices
120g/4oz	dwarf French/fine green or runner/green beans	1 cup
1 tbs	olive oil	1 tbs
1 large	onion, finely chopped	1 large
1 small	potato, diced	1 small
1	carrot, diced	1
1	stick/stalk celery, diced	1
1	courgette/zucchini, diced	1
230g/8oz	canned, chopped tomatoes	2 cups
1 tbs	chopped basil	1 tbs
1 tbs	chopped parsley	1 tbs
1 tbs	tomato purée/tomato paste	1 tbs
1l/1¾ pint	stock	4¼ cups
60g/2oz	small wholewheat pasta shapes or spaghetti broken into pieces	½ cup
60g/2oz	Parmesan cheese, finely grated	½ cup

1. Put the haricot beans (navy beans) into a bowl, cover with double their volume of cold water and leave to soak for 6–8 hours or overnight.
2. Drain the beans, rinse, drain again and then put them into a saucepan, cover with fresh cold water and bring to the boil. Boil rapidly for about 15 minutes. While preparing the vegetables leave to simmer gently.
3. Cut the dwarf French beans into 1 in lengths.
4. De-rind the bacon and cut it into 2cm (¾ in) wide strips.
5. Heat the oil in a large saucepan, add the onion and stir-fry for 3–4 minutes. Add the potato, carrot, celery, courgette (zucchini), bacon, tomatoes and herbs.
6. Blend the tomato purée (tomato paste) with the stock and stir into the vegetable mixture and dwarf French beans.
7. Drain the haricot beans (navy beans) and add them to the saucepan.
8. Bring the mixture to the boil, then cover and leave to simmer gently over a low heat for 1 hour 40 minutes.
9. Add the pasta to the simmering soup, stir well, then cover and simmer for about 15 minutes until the pasta is cooked.
10. Ladle the soup into warm bowls and sprinkle with the Parmesan cheese.

PARSNIP SOUP WITH APPLE

This thick, smooth soup contrasts well with the small cubes of crisp apple.

Serves 6

Metric/Imperial		American
15g/½ oz	margarine	1 tbs
1 large	onion, chopped	1 large
600g/1¼ lb	parsnips, roughly chopped	1¼ lb
7.5–10cm/3–4in	sprig of rosemary	3–4 in
600ml/1 pint	vegetable stock	2½ cups
240ml/8 fl oz	milk	1 cup
	lemon juice	
1	dessert/sweet apple, cored and diced	1

1. Melt the margarine in a saucepan, then add the onion and stir-fry for 3–4 minutes.
2. Add the parsnips, rosemary and stock and bring to the boil. Stir, cover the saucepan, reduce the heat and leave to simmer for 30–35 minutes.
3. Allow the soup to cool for a few minutes then remove the rosemary, leaving any unattached spiky leaves.
4. Transfer the vegetables and stock to a food process or liquidizer (blender) and blend to a purée.
5. Pour the purée back into the saucepan, stir in the milk and a little lemon juice.
6. Add the apple to the soup and stir over a low heat until the soup is steaming. Adjust the seasoning, adding a little more lemon juice to taste.

Fruit and vegetable recipes

POTATO SALAD

This recipe can be served hot or cold and the flavour can be varied by adjusting the quantities of herbs to suit your taste.

Serves 4

Metric/Imperial		*American*
450g/1lb	new potatoes	1 lb
150ml/5 fl oz	natural/plain yogurt	⅔ cup
1 tsp	finely chopped mint	1 tsp
1 tsp	finely chopped parsley	1 tsp
1 tsp	finely chopped chives	1 tsp

1. Scrub the potatoes and cook them in boiling water for about 15 minutes, then drain well and put into a bowl.
2. Mix the yogurt with the mint, parsley and chives.
3. Spoon the yogurt and herb dressing over the potatoes and mix well. Serve hot or cold.

Note to Cooks

Not suitable for freezing.

RATATOUILLE

If you can eat garlic without aggravating the symptoms of IBS, add 1 or 2 finely chopped cloves when the onions are cooked – they will enhance the flavour considerably. Although this recipe may be frozen, the texture of the vegetables diminishes a little when they are thawed and reheated.

Serves 4

Metric/Imperial		American
1 large or 2 small	aubergines/eggplants	1 large or 2 small
	salt	
1 small	sweet/red pepper	1 small
1 small	bell/green pepper	1 small
2 small	courgettes (zucchini)	2 small
2 tbs	olive oil	2 tbs
1 large	onion, roughly chopped	1 large
2	marmande/beefsteak tomatoes	2
1 tbs	chopped basil	1 tbs

1. Cut the aubergines (eggplants) into 2.5–4cm (1–1½ in) slices then cut each slice into quarters. Spread about half of the aubergines (eggplants) over the base of a colander or sieve (strainer), sprinkle them with salt, top with the remaining aubergines (eggplants) and sprinkle with a little more salt. Place the colander or sieve (strainer) over a bowl and leave for about 40 minutes to allow the bitter juices to drip away.

Fruit and vegetable recipes

2. Remove the cores and seeds from the peppers and cut into 2.5cm (1 in) squares. Cut the courgettes (zucchini) into 4cm (1½in) chunks.

3. Heat the oil in a large heavy-based saucepan, add the onion, stir round, then cover and leave over a low heat for 10 minutes.

4. Add the peppers, cover and leave for a further 5 minutes.

5. Rinse the aubergine (eggplant) very well under cold running water, pat dry then add to the saucepan with the courgettes (zucchini). Stir all the vegetables together, then cover the saucepan and leave for 30 minutes, stirring halfway through the cooking time.

6. Pour boiling water over the tomatoes, leave for 30–40 seconds then drain and slip off the skins. Cut each tomato into about 10 pieces.

7. Add the tomato and basil to the saucepan, stir well, cover and leave over a low heat until the vegetables are just cooked but still retain their shapes.

SAVOURY BANANA SALAD

Make this salad just a short while before serving, otherwise the watercress will wilt. If you prefer, substitute the sweetcorn with cooked frozen corn.

Serves 4

Metric/Imperial		American
1	banana	1
1 tsp	lemon juice	1 tsp
120g/4oz	canned sweetcorn, drained	⅔ cup
30g/1oz	watercress	1 cup
15g/½ oz	spring onions/scallions	3 medium
60g/2oz	curd cheese/ricotta	4 tbs
6 tbs	natural/plain yogurt	6 tbs

1. Peel and slice the banana into a bowl, add the lemon juice and sweetcorn and mix well.
2. Roughly chop the watercress and finely slice or chop the spring onions (scallions), then mix them into the banana mixture.
3. Spoon the curd cheese (ricotta) into a small bowl and gradually blend in the yogurt, a tbs at a time.
4. Spoon the curd cheese (ricotta) and yogurt dressing into the banana mixture and stir well.

Note to Cooks

Not suitable for freezing.

SIMPLE VEGETABLE SOUP

This soup is simple to make and uses ingredients that are often found in the store cupboard. Serve it with warm wholemeal (wholewheat) French bread or rolls.

Serves 4

Metric/Imperial		*American*
30g/1oz	margarine	2 tbs
180g/6oz	onion, chopped	1 medium
180g/6oz	potato, diced	1 medium
360g/12oz	sweetcorn, canned and drained or frozen	2 cups
2 × 230g/8oz	canned, chopped tomatoes	2 cups
600ml/1 pint	vegetable stock	2½ cups

1. Melt the margarine in a saucepan, add the onion, stir-fry for 1–2 minutes, then cover and leave over a low heat for 7–8 minutes.
2. Add the potatoes to the saucepan, together with the sweetcorn, tomatoes and stock. Cover and simmer for about 30 minutes.
3. Ladle the soup into 4 warm serving bowls.

SPRINGTIME SALAD

Sprinkle toasted oatmeal over the salad just before serving so it remains deliciously crunchy.

Serves 4

Metric/Imperial		American
120g/4oz	large, black grapes	1 cup
1 large	banana	1 large
¼	galia or canteloupe melon	¼
180g/6oz	fromage frais	¾ cup
1 tbs	clear honey	1 tbs
45g/1½oz	porridge oats	⅜ cup

1. Cut the grapes in half, remove the pips (seeds) and put the grape halves into a bowl.
2. Peel and thickly slice the banana and add to the grapes.
3. Remove the seeds from the melon, cut away the skin, then cut the flesh into 1.25cm (½ in) cubes.
4. Mix all the fruits together then spoon them into 4 serving glasses.
5. Just before serving, mix the fromage frais with the honey. Spread the porridge oats evenly on a baking tray (baking sheet). Cook the oats under a hot grill (broiler), shaking the tray (sheet) gently every so often until they are all brown but not burnt.
6. Spoon the fromage frais on top of each fruit salad, sprinkle the toasted oats over the top and serve.

Note to Cooks

Not suitable for freezing.

Fruit and vegetable recipes

STIR-FRIED VEGETABLES

By following the method below the vegetables will be piping hot but they will still retain their shape and texture.

Serves 4

Metric/Imperial		American
8	spring onions/scallions	8
1 small	sweet/red pepper	1 small
1	courgette/zucchini	1
180g/6oz	cauliflower and broccoli florets	1½ cups
60g/2oz	button mushrooms	1 cup
1 tbs	sesame oil	1 tbs
60g/2oz	fennel bulb, thinly sliced	⅔ cup
90g/3oz	beansprouts	1½ cups
2–2½ tbs	soy/soya sauce	2–2½ tbs
1 tbs	lemon juice	1 tbs

1. Cut the spring onions (scallions) into 2.5cm (1 in) lengths.
2. Deseed the pepper then cut it into 2.5cm (1 in) strips about 6mm (¼ in) wide. Cut the courgette (zucchini) into the same sized lengths.
3. Cut the stalks from the cauliflower and broccoli. Chop the stalks but leave the tiny florets whole.
4. If the mushrooms are very small, leave them whole, otherwise halve or slice them.

5. Heat the oil in a wok or heavy-based saucepan until it is very hot, then add the onions and stir-fry for 1 minute.
6. Add the pepper, fennel, cauliflower and broccoli and stir-fry for 3–4 minutes.
7. Add the courgettes (zucchini), mushrooms and beansprouts and stir round for 1 minute.
8. Add 2 tbs of the soy/soya sauce and the lemon juice and cook for a further minute. Adjust the seasoning to taste by adding a little more soy/soya sauce if necessary, then serve immediately.

Note to Cooks

Not suitable for freezing.

STUFFED MUSHROOMS

Use very lean cooked ham for this recipe.

Serves 4

Metric/Imperial		*American*
4 large	field/flat cap mushrooms	4 large
15g/½ oz	margarine	1 tbs
30g/1oz	onion, finely chopped	1 small
90g/3oz	fresh wholemeal/	1½ cups
	wholewheat breadcrumbs	
60g/2oz	cooked ham, finely chopped	3 slices
30g/1oz	smoked hard cheese,	¼ cup
	coarsely grated	
1	egg, beaten	1
4 slices	wholemeal/wholewheat	4 slices
	toast	

1. Remove the stalks from the mushrooms and finely chop them.
2. Melt the margarine in a saucepan, add the onion and mushroom stalks and stir-fry for 4–5 minutes or until the moisture, which runs from the mushrooms, has evaporated, then remove the pan from the heat.
3. Stir the breadcrumbs, ham and cheese into the mushroom mixture.
4. Add the beaten egg and stir round to bind all the stuffing ingredients.
5. Spoon the stuffing evenly into the mushroom caps then put them into a lightly greased ovenproof dish,

cover with foil and bake at 400°F/200°C/gas mark 6 for 15–16 minutes. (Do not overcook or the liquid will start to ooze from them.)

6. Serve the Stuffed Mushrooms with the slices of toast.

Note to Cooks

Not suitable for freezing.

STUFFED TOMATOES

Serve these tomatoes on a bed of shredded lettuce leaves, accompanied by a selection of salads.

Serves 3

Metric/Imperial		American
3 × 300g/10oz	marmande/beefsteak tomatoes	3 large
	salt	
90g/3oz	long-grain brown rice	scant ½ cup
240g/8oz	boil-in-the-bag kipper fillets	2
2 tsp	olive oil	2 tsp
3½ tbs	spring onions/scallions, finely chopped	3½ tbs

1. Cut and remove a 12mm (½ in) slice from the top of each tomato. Scoop out and discard the seeds, or add them to the saucepan when making tomato sauce. Carefully remove then chop the fleshly dividing walls between the tomato seeds.
2. Sprinkle the inside of each tomato liberally with salt, turn them upside down, and lay in a colander or sieve (strainer) to draw out the excess water. Leave them for 30 minutes. Rinse them well under cold running water then pat dry with kitchen paper (paper towels).
3. Cook the rice according to the instructions on the packet until the grains are fluffy and separate.

4. Cook the kipper fillets according to the instructions on the packet, then flake onto a plate, removing any bones.
5. Heat the oil in a small saucepan, add the spring onions (scallions) and stir-fry for 2–3 minutes. Add the chopped pieces of tomato and stir over a low heat for about 5 minutes until the tomato pulp reduces to form a thick purée.
6. Mix the rice with the kipper, spring onions (scallions) and tomato mixture.
7. Spoon the rice stuffing into the tomatoes and replace the tomato tops. Put the Stuffed Tomatoes onto a baking tray (baking sheet) and bake at 350°F/ 180°C/ gas mark 4 for 25–30 minutes.

Note to Cooks

Not suitable for freezing.

SUMMER SALAD

This recipe illustrates how a variety of salads can be served together to provide a meal that consists of several textures, flavours and colours yet is relatively low in fat and calories.

Serves 1

Metric/Imperial		*American*
60g/2oz	cottage/pot cheese	¼ cup
60g/2oz	fromage frais	¼ cup
70g/2½oz	dessert/sweet apple	½
1 tsp	chives, chopped	1 tsp
1 portion	Potato Salad (see page 172)	1 portion
1 portion	Fruity Beetroot (see page 167)	1 portion
1 portion	Cucumber Salad (see page 162)	1 portion
	Few sprigs watercress to garnish	

1. Mix the cottage (pot) cheese with the fromage frais.
2. Core and quarter the apple, then cut it into small dice. Stir the apple and chives into the cheese and fromage frais mixture.
3. Spoon the cheese and apple mixture onto a large serving plate, surround it with the other salads, then garnish with the sprigs of watercress.

Note to Cooks

Not suitable for freezing.

SWEETCORN AND PEAS

This tasty recipe is an ideal accompaniment to an elaborate main course or a simple omelette.

Serves 4

Metric/Imperial		American
90–120g/3–4oz	lean bacon	4 slices
2 tsp	oil	2 tsp
1 small	onion, finely chopped	1 small
150g/5oz	frozen sweetcorn	1 cup
90g/3oz	frozen petit pois	½ cup
5 tbs	tomato juice	5 tbs
90g/3oz	quark	6 tbs

1. Derind the bacon and cut it into short strips.
2. Heat the oil in a saucepan, add the onion and stir-fry until it becomes translucent.
3. Add the bacon strips and stir over a low heat for 2–3 minutes.
4. Tip the sweetcorn and petit pois into the saucepan, stir in the tomato juice and bring to the boil. Reduce the heat as low as possible and leave to barely simmer for 6–7 minutes.
5. Stir the vegetables, add the quark and leave over the low heat until it has melted then serve immediately.

Note to Cooks

Not suitable for freezing.

VEGETABLE BARLEY CASSEROLE

This recipe may be cooked on a very low heat on the stove instead of baking, but stir it occasionally to prevent it burning.

Serves 6

Metric/Imperial		American
180g/6oz	leek	1 large
2	sticks/stalk celery	2
300g/10oz	carrots and parsnips, swedes/rutabagas and turnips/turnip roots	2 cups
120g/4oz	button mushrooms	2 cups
2 tsp	oil	2 tsp
120g/4oz	fennel bulb, sliced	1 cup
90g/3oz	peas	½ cup
180g/6oz	pearl/pot barley	¾ cup
2 tbs	chopped parsley	2 tbs
1 tbs	tomato purée/tomato paste	1 tbs
600ml/1 pint	vegetable stock	2½ cups

1. Cut the leek and celery into thick slices.
2. Cut the carrots, parsnips, swede (rutabaga) and turnips (turnip roots) into 12mm (½ in) cubes.
3. Quarter the button mushrooms.
4. Heat the oil in an ovenproof casserole, add the slices of leek and stir-fry for 2–3 minutes. Stir in the remaining vegetables, pearl barley (pot barley) and parsley.

5. Mix the tomato purée (tomato paste) and stock together in a jug, then stir into the casserole. Bring to the boil, stir well, cover and bake in a moderate oven (350°F/180°C/gas mark 4) for 50–60 minutes until the stock has been absorbed and the vegetables are tender.

WHOLE TOMATO SALAD

These stuffed tomatoes make an appetizing addition to a main course but could also be served as an hors-d'oeuvre.

Serves 4

Metric/Imperial		American
4	marmande/beefsteak tomatoes	4
	salt	
90g/3oz	long-grain rice	⅜ cup
45g/1½oz	cucumber, finely chopped	2 in piece
45g/1½oz	spring onions/scallions, finely chopped	5 large
2–3 tbs	mayonnaise	2–3 tbs

1. Cut a slice from the top of each tomato and put it to one side. Scoop out and discard all the seeds, then carefully scrape out the ridges of tomato flesh and chop them. Put the chopped tomato in a sieve (strainer) to allow the liquid to drain from it.
2. Turn the tomatoes upside down in a colander or sieve (strainer) for about 30 minutes and leave to drain.
3. Cook the rice as directed on the packet until the grains are fluffy and separate, then leave to cool.
4. Mix the drained chopped tomato with the rice, cucumber and spring onions (scallions), then stir in the mayonnaise.
5. Spoon the rice mixture into each tomato skin and put the tomato tops back on top of the tomatoes.

Note to Cooks
Not suitable for freezing.

Irritable Bowel Syndrome

BRAMBLE BROWN BETTY

Serve this dish with yogurt or plain fromage frais.

Serves 6

Metric/Imperial		American
840g/1¾ lb	cooking/tart apples	1¾ lb
180g/6oz	wholemeal/wholewheat breadcrumbs	3 cups
60g/2oz	soft brown sugar	⅓ cup
240g/8oz	blackberries	2 cups
15g/½ oz	margarine	1 tbs

1. Peel, quarter then core and thinly slice the apples.
2. Stir the breadcrumbs with the sugar.
3. Spoon a third of the breadcrumb mixture evenly over the bottom of a lightly greased deep ovenproof dish, approximately 17.5cm (7 in) in diameter.
4. Arrange half the apple slices on top of the bread-crumbs, then scatter about half the blackberries over them. Sprinkle another third of the breadcrumbs over the fruit and layer the remaining breadcrumbs and fruit in the same order.
5. Dot the margarine over the breadcrumbs then bake at 350°F/180°C/gas mark 4 for about 50 minutes until the fruit is tender and the topping crisp and golden brown.

CREAMY-TOPPED FRUIT

This creamy topping tastes good over a variety of fruits.

Serves 4

Metric/Imperial		American
60g/2oz	curd cheese/ricotta	¼ cup
120g/4oz	fromage frais	½ cup
2 tsp	honey	2 tsp
1 tsp	lemon zest, finely grated	1 tsp
120g/4oz	kumquats	1 cup
8	fresh dates	8
120g/4oz	pineapple, fresh or canned and drained	1 cup
1	banana	1
2 tsp	lemon juice	2 tsp

1. Mash the curd cheese (ricotta) with a fork then gradually add the fromage frais and combine well to form a thick, smooth mixture. Stir in the honey and lemon zest and put the mixture into the refrigerator.
2. Halve the kumquats, halve and stone (pit) the dates and cut the pineapple into pieces the same size as the kumquats.
3. Peel and cut the banana into thick slices and toss them in the lemon juice.
4. Mix all the fruit together then spoon into 4 serving glasses and spoon the chilled topping over. Refrigerate for 1–2 hours.

Note to Cooks
Not suitable for freezing.

DRIED FRUIT COMPOTE

This compote can be made at any time of the year and you can alter the proportions of one fruit, making sure you have the same overall weight, to suit your taste. It makes a delicious dessert but is also a refreshing breakfast dish.

Serves 6

Metric/Imperial		American
30g/1oz	dried apple rings	2 tsp
60g/1oz	dried peaches	⅓ cup
60g/2oz	dried apricots	⅓ cup
60g/2oz	dried figs, quartered	⅓ cup
60g/2oz	dried stoned/pitted prunes	⅓ cup
450ml/¾ pint	orange juice	2 cups

1. Put all the dried fruits into a bowl, cover with the orange juice and leave to soak for several hours or overnight.
2. Pour the soaked fruits and orange juice into a saucepan and heat gently until it is barely simmering. Cover and leave for 10–15 minutes. Serve hot or chilled.

FRESH FRUIT JELLY

Unlike a lot of brightly coloured jellies sold in shops, this jelly is full of real fruit. The amount of sugar will vary depending on the sweetness of the fruit.

Serves 4

Metric/Imperial		American
120ml/4 fl oz	grape or orange juice	½ cup
1 sachet	gelatine	1½ level tbs
180g/6oz	strawberries	1½ cups
240g/8oz	canned pineapple chunks in their own juice	1 cup
½–1½ tsp	caster/superfine sugar	½–1½ tsp

To serve

360g/12oz	strawberries	3 cups

1. Pour 3 tbs of the grape or orange juice into a small bowl or cup, sprinkle in the gelatine, stir well and stand in a saucepan of simmering water until the gelatine granules have completely dissolved.
2. Pour the remaining grape or orange juice, together with the strawberries, pineapple and its juice and sugar into a liquidizer (blender). Process until it forms a smooth purée.
3. Stir the juice and gelatine mixture thoroughly into the fruit purée then pour it into a 600ml (1 pint/2½ cup) ring mould (tube pan) and chill for a few hours until it has set. (*Note* it will take longer than a commercial jelly.)

4. Dip the mould briefly into hot water then invert it onto the serving plate and the jelly should come out cleanly. Made like this, the jelly will be cloudy, but clear on top. If you want the colour and fruit to be evenly distributed, stir the jelly well when it is half set.
5. Fill the centre of the jelly ring with the fresh strawberries.

FRUIT BARS

These chewy bars can be eaten at breakfast, for dessert or cut into pieces and handed round as sweets.

Serves 4

Metric/Imperial		American
60g/2oz	raisins	6 tbs
60g/2oz	stoned/pitted dried dates, chopped	⅛ cup
60g/2oz	dried apricots, roughly chopped	⅛ cup
30g/1oz	hazelnut kernels	¼ cup
30g/1oz	ground almonds	¼ cup
2–3 tsp	lemon juice	2–3 tsp
	rice paper	

1. Put the raisins, dates, apricots and nuts into a liquidizer (blender) and process for a few seconds.
2. Add the ground almonds and 2 tsp of the lemon juice and process once again until it forms a moist mixture that *just* sticks together (if it is too dry add a little more lemon juice).
3. Spoon the mixture onto a piece of rice paper and, using the back of a spoon or a palette knife (narrow spatula), spread it into a rectangle about 10 × 12cm (4 × 4½ in).
4. Transfer the fruit slab to the refrigerator and chill for 2–3 hours, then cut the mixture into 4 bars and refrigerate until required. These bars will keep for up to 3 days in the refrigerator.

FRUITELS

These tasty sweets (candies) are an ideal substitute for traditional confectionery.

Makes 12, Serves 4

Metric/Imperial		American
45g/1½oz	hazelnuts, roasted	⅜cup
60g/2oz	currants	3 tbs
60g/2oz	raisins	6 tbs
60g/2oz	sultanas/golden seedless raisins	⅓ cup

1. Put all but a quarter of the hazelnuts into a liquidizer (blender). Add the dried fruit and process to a thick, sticky pulp. (It may be necessary to stop the liquidizer (blender) and draw the fruit and nuts up before continuing to blend as the mixture tends to stick round the blades.)
2. Finely chop the reserved hazelnuts then spread them evenly on a plate.
3. Spoon a heaped tsp of the fruit and nut mixture onto the nuts and, using your hands, roll until it forms a ball and is coated with nuts. Continue until all the ingredients have been used.
4. Transfer the Fruitels to a clean plate and refrigerate for about 30 minutes until firm.

FRUITY CHEESE RING

This recipe makes an attractive dessert for a dinner party. If you don't have a ring mould (tube pan) set the mousse in a plain one and arrange the fruit around the edge of it.

Serves 6

Metric/Imperial		American
90g/3oz	no-soak dried apricots	1 cup
240g/8oz	ricotta cheese	1 cup
150ml/¼ pint	milk	⅔ cup
30g/1oz	caster/superfine sugar	2 tbs
2 tbs	lemon juice	2 tbs
	few drops of vanilla essence/ vanilla extract	
1 sachet	gelatine	1½ level tbs
120g/4oz	strawberries	1 cup
120g/4oz	kumquats	1 cup

1. Roughly chop the apricots then place in a small saucepan. Add 8 tbs water, cover the saucepan and leave to simmer for 15 minutes over a very low heat. Leave to cool.
2. Put the ricotta, milk, sugar and lemon juice into a liquidizer (blender) and process until smooth.
3. Drain the apricots, reserving the cooking liquid, and add them to the liquidizer (blender). Add a few drops of vanilla essence (vanilla extract) to taste. Process once again until the mixture is smooth.

4. Spoon the cooking liquid from the apricots into a small cup or bowl and, if necessary, make up to 2–3 tbs of liquid with a little water. Sprinkle the gelatine into the liquid and put the cup or bowl into a saucepan of simmering water until the gelatine has dissolved.

5. Pour the gelatine mixture into the liquidizer (blender) and process the mixture again until it is well combined. Then pour it into a 750ml (1¼ pint/⅝ quart) ring mould (tube pan) and chill until it has set.

6. To serve, dip the mould briefly in hot water and invert it onto a serving plate, tap sharply and lift the mould away from the apricot cheese mixture.

7. Slice the strawberries and halve or quarter the kumquats, pile the fruit in the centre of the ring and serve.

OATMEAL AMBROSIA

If you prefer, substitute the apricots with other dried fruits.

Serves 3

Metric/Imperial		*American*
90g/3oz	dried apricots	½ cup
180ml/6 fl oz	orange juice	¾ cup
30g/1oz	porridge oats	¼ cup
150ml/¼ pint	milk	⅔ cup
Approx.	honey	Approx.
4 tsp		4 tsp
120g/4oz	fromage frais	½ cup

1. Chop the apricots and put them in a non-metallic bowl.
2. Heat the orange juice until it is steaming, then pour it over the apricots and leave them to soak for several hours or, preferably, overnight.
3. Put all but a heaped tbs of the apricots with the orange juice into a liquidizer (blender) and process thoroughly to form a slightly chunky purée.
4. Spoon the porridge oats into a small saucepan, add the milk and bring to the boil, stirring all the time. Stir the fruit purée into the saucepan and continue to boil, gently stirring, continuously for 3–4 minutes until the mixture becomes thick.
5. Remove the saucepan from the heat, sweeten with a little honey to taste and leave the mixture to cool.
6. Stir in the reserved apricots and fromage frais.
7. Spoon the Oatmeal Ambrosia into 3 serving glasses and leave until cold.

PEACHES WITH RASPBERRIES

This dish is very refreshing and is particularly welcome on a hot summer's day when the fruits are in season and full of flavour.

Serves 2

Metric/Imperial		American
120g/4oz	raspberries	1 cup
90g/3oz	fromage frais	¾ cup
½–1 tsp	caster/superfine sugar	½–1 tsp
½–1 tsp	lemon juice	½–1 tsp
2 large	peaches or nectarines	2 large

1. Put the raspberries and fromage frais into a liquidizer (blender) and process for a few seconds.
2. Pour the raspberry and fromage frais mixture into a small bowl, stir in the sugar and lemon juice to taste, then refrigerate for about 20 minutes to thicken the sauce.
3. Just before serving, cut the peaches or nectarines in half and remove the stones (pits). Put 2 halves on each serving dish and spoon over the raspberry sauce.

Note to Cooks

Not suitable for freezing.

STUFFED APPLES

Adjust the amount of honey according to the sweetness of the cooking (tart) apples.

Serves 4

Metric/Imperial		American
4 × 240–270g/ 8–9oz	cooking/tart apples	4 medium
45g/1½oz	dried mixed fruit	¼ cup
2–4 tsp	honey	2–4 tsp

1. Core the apples, cutting about 12mm (½ in) from the bottom end of each core. Replace these in each apple to prevent the filling from falling out.
2. Score around the centre of each apple to help prevent it splitting during cooking.
3. Mix the dried fruit with the honey.
4. Stand the apples in an ovenproof dish and spoon a quarter of the honey and dried fruit mixture into each one.
5. Pour 4 tbs water into the dish and bake at 350°F/ 180°C/gas mark 4 for about 50 minutes until the apples are just soft.

Note to Cooks

Not suitable for freezing.

SUMMER SUNDAE

Use really fresh, ripe fruit for this recipe so it not only tastes good, but looks good!

Serves 2

Metric/Imperial		American
240g/8oz	apricots	2 cups
120g/4oz	raspberries	1 cup
90g/3oz	curd cheese/ricotta	6 tbs
1 tsp	caster/superfine sugar	1 tsp
	few drops of vanilla essence/ vanilla extract	
2 tbs	low-fat natural/plain yogurt	2 tbs

1. Halve the apricots, remove the stones (pits) and roughly chop the flesh.
2. Spoon half the raspberries and all the apricots into 2 serving glasses.
3. Using a fork, mix the curd cheese (ricotta), sugar, vanilla and yogurt together until you have a smooth cream.
4. Mash the remaining raspberries to a purée. Stir the raspberry purée unevenly into the curd cheese (ricotta) and yogurt mixture then spoon it on top of the apricots and raspberries.

Note to Cooks

Not suitable for freezing.

SWEET DATE PANCAKES (CRÊPES)

If you wish to serve these pancakes (crêpes) during a dinner or lunch party, make the batter and cook the pancakes (crêpes) well ahead of time then cover loosely with foil and reheat in a warm oven. Mix the filling ingredients together and then complete the recipe just before serving.

Serves 6

Metric/Imperial		American
1 quantity	Pancake (Crêpe) Batter (see page 149)	1 quantity
180g/6oz	curd cheese/ricotta finely grated zest and juice of ½ an orange	¾ cup
4 tsp	orange juice	4 tsp
1 tsp	caster/superfine sugar	1 tsp
180g/6oz	fresh dates	6 medium

1. Make the Pancake (Crêpe) Batter and cook as described on page 149.
2. Mix the curd cheese (ricotta) together with the orange zest, juice and sugar.
3. Stone (pit) and finely chop the dates.
4. Spread a spoonful of the curd cheese (ricotta) mixture over each pancake (crêpe), sprinkle with the chopped dates then either roll up or fold in quarters and serve.

Note to Cooks

Not suitable for freezing.

WINTER FRUIT SALAD

This salad incorporates fruits that are available during the winter months.

Serves 4

Metric/Imperial		American
1	apple	1
6	fresh dates	6
1	mandarin	1
1	banana	1
6 tbs	natural/plain yogurt	6 tbs
	lemon juice	
30g/1oz	Breakfast Crunch (see page 93)	2 heaped tbs

1. Core the apple, cut it into quarters, then chunks and place in a bowl.
2. Stone (pit) the dates, then cut them into quarters and add to the apple.
3. Peel the mandarin, divide it into segments and add to the apple and dates.
4. Just before serving, mash the banana with the yogurt until it is smooth, then add lemon juice to taste.
5. Spoon the banana and yogurt mixture into the bowl with the fruits and stir well. Add the Breakfast Crunch and mix once again.
6. Spoon the Winter Fruit Salad into 4 serving glasses or dishes and serve immediately.

Note to Cooks
Not suitable for freezing.

Fruit and vegetable recipes

Further Reading

Coultate, T., and Davies, J., Food: The Definitive Guide, Royal Society of Chemistry, 1994

Davies, J., and Dickerson, J., Nutrient Content of Food Portions, Royal Society of Chemistry, 1991.

Department of Health, Dietary Reference Values for Food Energy and Nutrients for the United Kingdom, H.M.S.O., 1991.

Heaton, K.W., Understanding your Bowels, BMA Family Doctor Series, 1993.

Janowitz, H.D., Your Gut Feelings, Prevention and Cure of Intestinal Problems, Oxford University Press, 1989.

Useful Addresses

British Digestive Foundation
3 St Andrew's Place
London NW1 4LB

The British Digestive Foundation exists to:

- Fund new research projects into digestive diseases
- Help sufferers with, for example practical guidelines on controlling their symptoms
- Provide information for the public

The leaflet on IBS produced by the British Digestive Foundation is particularly useful for sufferers.

The IBS Appeal (L)
Central Middlesex Hospital
NHS Trust
Acton Lane
London NW10 7NS

The IBS Appeal has a research team investigating the causes of IBS with the aim of developing cures. A quarterly bulletin reports on the latest progress of other research teams throughout the world.

IBS Network
Centre for Human Nutrition
Northern General Hospital
Sheffield S5 7AU

The IBS Network has a network of self help groups and produces a quarterly newsletter called GUT Reaction. The newsletter is by IBS sufferers for IBS sufferers.

Centre for Bowel Research
South Bank University
103 Borough Road
London SE1 0AA

The Centre for Bowel Research at South Bank University is carrying out studies into 'normal' parameters of bowel function and bowel disorders including constipation and irritable bowel syndrome. If you would like to participate in the research contact Dr Jill Davies.

Index

Index of Recipes

Irritable Bowel Syndrome